Confronting Chronic Pain

CONFRONTING CHRONIC PAIN

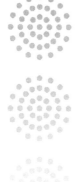

A Pain Doctor's Guide to Relief

STEVEN H. RICHEIMER, M.D.
with
KATHY STELIGO

JOHNS HOPKINS UNIVERSITY PRESS
Baltimore

Note to the Reader. This book is not meant to substitute for medical care of people with pain, and treatment should not be based solely on its contents. Instead, treatment must be developed in a dialogue between the individual and his or her physician. Our book has been written to help with that dialogue.

Drug dosage: The author and publisher have made reasonable efforts to determine that the selection of drugs discussed in this text conform to the practices of the general medical community. The medications described do not necessarily have specific approval by the U.S. Food and Drug Administration for use in the diseases for which they are recommended. In view of ongoing research, changes in governmental regulations, and the constant flow of information relating to drug therapy and drug reactions, the reader is urged to check the package insert of each drug for any change in indications and dosage and for warnings and precautions. This is particularly important when the recommended agent is a new and/or infrequently used drug.

© 2014 Johns Hopkins University Press
All rights reserved. Published 2014
Printed in the United States of America on acid-free paper
9 8 7 6 5 4 3 2 1

Johns Hopkins University Press
2715 North Charles Street
Baltimore, Maryland 21218-4363
www.press.jhu.edu

Library of Congress Cataloging-in-Publication Data

Richeimer, Steven, author.
　Confronting Chronic Pain : a pain doctor's guide to relief / Steven H. Richeimer, M.D. ; with Kathy Steligo.
　　　pages cm. — (A Johns Hopkins Press health book)
　Includes bibliographical references and index.
　ISBN-13: 978-1-4214-1252-8 (hardcover : alk. paper)
　ISBN-10: 1-4214-1252-7 (hardcover : alk. paper)
　ISBN-13: 978-1-4214-1253-5 (pbk. : alk. paper)
　ISBN-10: 1-4214-1253-5 (pbk. : alk. paper)
　ISBN-13: 978-1-4214-1254-2 (electronic)
　ISBN-10: 1-4214-1254-3 (electronic)
　1. Chronic pain—Popular works. 2. Analgesia—Popular works. 3. Mind and body therapies. I. Steligo, Kathy. II. Title.
　RB127.R528 2014
　615.8'52—dc23　　　　2013021126

A catalog record for this book is available from the British Library.

Special discounts are available for bulk purchases of this book. For more information, please contact Special Sales at 410-516-6936 or specialsales@press.jhu.edu.

Johns Hopkins University Press uses environmentally friendly book materials, including recycled text paper that is composed of at least 30 percent post-consumer waste, whenever possible.

Contents

Tables

Foreword

Chronic pain can change your life or the life of a loved one; if you are reading this book, it has probably already done so. Pain, the body's danger signal of potential or actual tissue damage, is an acute neurophysiological event in the central nervous system, but pain can become a chronic condition that reverberates in our minds and emotions and profoundly alters our lives. Chronic pain is so common and affects so many lives that it seems impossible for any of us to be so isolated from others that we would be unaware of pain's impact. How *you* learn to manage chronic pain, and how *you* manage the physicians and other practitioners caring for you affects how life will turn out for you. Given the right tools for self-management and the right health care team providing a personalized combination of appropriate treatments, most people with chronic pain do quite well over time and even grow during the experience. I can say this with some confidence after devoting 30 years to the problem of understanding and helping patients manage chronic or recurrent pain and teaching others how to do this.

Pain may call to action the best features of our profit-driven health care system. It is a system of phenomenal ability, yet when we try to manage persistent pain, the functionality of our health system often shifts toward dysfunction and disarray. Embedded in a hunt-find-cure training perspective and undereducated about changes in the brain and the spinal cord that perpetuate pain, doctors may persist in seeking a possible cause or cure through tests, procedures, and surgeries while they overlook the patient's suffering and deterioration. This pursuit is reinforced by an entire system that is organized to reward utilization of technology and procedures rather than focusing on maximizing patients' health, happiness, function, and quality of life. It is during this often futile search that pain's damage to the nervous system begins and a person's life begins to change. Our population faces significant challenges regarding pain: the dire need for better training of our health care workforce and for greatly expanded research to find better, safer treatment.

It may be hard to believe that pain can help you grow, but this unique, wonderful book by Steven Richeimer and Kathy Steligo will give you hope and a navigational chart for getting better. With easily understood prose, helpful tables and illustrations, and convincing case histories, they explain how you can cope and grow through understanding the ways your body, mind, and spirit work together in healing. The authors do not promise miracles. Instead, they call on your own potential, using what we know about chronic pain and its treatments and using your own spiritual resources, to learn how to manage pain effectively and to reduce your personal suffering. Their guide will help you (or a loved one) reverse the downward trajectory of chronic pain and change the outcome of your (or your loved one's) life.

Dr. Richeimer, currently a professor and director of pain medicine at the University of Southern California, is one our nation's leading pain-medicine specialists. Endowed with education and training from leading universities such as Stanford University, the University of California–Los Angeles, the University of California–San Francisco, and Harvard University, he also holds credentials in anesthesiology, psychiatry, and the new specialty of pain medicine. His most important credential, however, is years of experience in using this training to care for patients with the most difficult and challenging chronic pain conditions, learning from them about their needs and how to best help them, and training others to this calling. Ms. Steligo, a skilled and experienced patient-education specialist, has written popular books that have helped people learn how to manage their lives with severe illnesses, such as breast cancer. These authors combine their talents admirably in this book. In this exceptional resource, the authors explain that when pain persists, it changes the way people think about themselves and the way their nervous system (the spinal cord and brain, where reflexes, thoughts, and emotions reside and direct behavior) functions. Pain is profoundly personal and private, resounding in our consciousness and in our suffering. Nowhere in medicine is empathy, a capacity to understand suffering in others, more needed but so difficult to sustain.

Although the science of pain is riveting—at least to those of us who call ourselves "painiacs" because we zealously attempt to understand pain and help those suffering from it—the science does not account for the other dimension in healing that Richeimer and Steligo address so poignantly in their book: the meaning of pain and our spiritual response. A discussion of this dimension is critical to coping with pain and healing from its effects on our lives, yet it is difficult to dissect or scientifically analyze and tends to be absent in medical journals or forums. Richeimer and Steligo address this issue head on, explaining the important distinction between pain and suffering and the critical need to tend to your spiritual self while living with pain.

This book is your road map for managing your pain and attaining a better quality of life. It calls on you to address all dimensions of your chronic pain: mind, body, spirit. Use it as a guide to understand the wide array of pain tools available and to work with your physician and health care team. Most important, let it guide you to a deeper appreciation of your own potential for managing your pain, for minimizing your suffering, and for healing.

Rollin M. Gallagher, M.D., M.P.H.
Director for Pain Policy Research and Primary Care,
    Penn Pain Medicine
Clinical Professor of Psychiatry and Anesthesiology,
    University of Pennsylvania
Deputy National Program Director for
    Pain Management, Veterans Health System
Board of Directors, American Academy of
    Pain Medicine
Editor-in-Chief, *Pain Medicine*

Acknowledgments

Throughout my life and career, I have been blessed with profoundly rewarding relationships. I cherish these individuals' counsel and friendship, and I am deeply indebted for the influence they have bestowed upon my personal and professional life: Dr. Philip Lumb, Chair of the Department of Anesthesiology at the University of Southern California, who has championed my work for more than a decade; Dr. Vladimir Zelman, our vice chair at USC; and Dr. Carol Warfield, chief of the Harvard-Beth Israel Pain Program when I was a fellow. All of you have touched my life, shaped my learning, and influenced my passion for helping people live better lives despite their pain.

I am also grateful to colleagues who have been friends and sounding boards for the past 20 years: Drs. Scott Fishman and Zahid Bajwa, and Dr. Rollin (Mac) Gallagher, my mentor in the world of clinical publishing.

I am privileged to work each day with a team of compassionate and knowledgeable clinicians and colleagues who care deeply about the welfare of our patients and make my job easier: Drs. Susan Axtell, Jack Berger, Rahki Dayal, Margaret Miller, Linda Rever, Michael Sniderman, Natalie Strand, and Faye Weinstein; Pamela Merriam, NP; and our staff: Monique Rodriquez, Ana Gerardo, Connie Vargas, and Corin Michel.

To each of the individuals who generously wrote about their personal experiences with pain for this text, I am very grateful. You know firsthand how difficult a life in constant pain can be. But you are also a testimony to the possibility of living a better and more fulfilling life, even when that pain persists. It is not always easy to share these intimate and sometimes complex experiences, and I am grateful for your willingness to share so that others can benefit from your experiences.

My love and appreciation go to my entire family for their love and support: my devoted wife Hilary, my wise parents Harvey and Eva; my children, Aliza and her husband Josh, Zack, Rebecca, and Joseph. Also to my sister Yvonne and my brother Alan, with whom I have had breakfast every Sunday for more than a decade. I give thanks for all of you each day.

Lastly, I am enormously grateful to Jacqueline Wehmueller, Executive Editor at Johns Hopkins University Press, for understanding the need for this book and for giving me the opportunity to share the possibility of a happy and joyful life with so many who are held captive to their pain.

May this book provide tools, insights, and healing to all of those in pain.

Steven H. Richeimer, M.D.

Introduction

"There is nothing we can do."

"You just have to live with it."

If you suffer with chronic pain, you may have repeatedly heard these disheartening words, but only in rare cases are they accurate.

Chronic pain appears in many forms. It may develop from damage to the spine, sending excruciating pain down the arms or the legs, or manifest as debilitating headaches that strike without pattern and last for days. In some people it occurs as extreme tenderness and aching throughout the body without apparent cause. While the sources of these various ailments may differ, one aspect remains constant: moderate to severe pain can have life-changing consequences that are impossible to understand for those without firsthand experience. Left untreated (or treated ineffectively), pervasive pain can prevent many of the essential movements most of us take for granted: standing, sitting, and lifting can be unbearable, and routine activities such as shopping for groceries, working, or caring for home and family become impossible. Depression develops, sleep becomes difficult, and emotional isolation occurs as people in pain withdraw from family and friends. Life unravels. Unchecked or uncontrolled, the cumulative effects of living with unrelenting pain can erode all aspects of an otherwise healthy life, creating physical, psychological, and social problems and spiritual vulnerability.

The World Health Organization identifies pain as one of the most underestimated global health care problems. In 2011, the Institute of Medicine (the independent health panel for the National Academy of Sciences) released *Relieving Pain in America: A Blueprint for Transforming Prevention, Care, Education, and Research,* a landmark report showing that pain is not well understood or optimally managed. Pain is so common that it is now considered as the fifth vital sign; hospitals assess it along with a patient's temperature, pulse, respiratory rate, and blood pressure. In the United States, the size of the affected community is staggering: an estimated 100 million people—more than all those with cancer, diabetes, and heart disease combined. The yearly cost in treatments and lost productivity is estimated at $635 billion, or nearly $2,000 for every person living in the United States.[1] The economic toll of chronic pain is monumental; the personal suffering it causes is immeasurable.

Despite the scope of the chronic pain problem, a chasm exists between a person's need for pain management and the medical establishment's ability to deliver that care. Although chronic pain is the most common reason people see a doctor and take pain medication, its subjective nature makes it difficult to diagnose and treat. Most chronic pain sufferers are treated by primary physicians whose medical training prepares them to find and fix disease but barely scratches the surface of pain management. Without appropriate training or experience, the average physician is ill equipped to understand the complexities of treating chronic pain, through no fault of his own. Half of all primary care doctors, the first line of defense for most people in pain, say they feel only "somewhat prepared" to help their patients with pain; about one-fourth of doctors feel "somewhat" or "very" unprepared.[2] With all of our advances, the average person in pain is often handed a bottle of Vicodin and sent home. Most suffer needlessly as they avoid taking the medication because of its side effects or live with the mistaken notion that "toughing it out" provides the best medical outcome, which is never the case. So it is easy to understand why, for many people, the quest for relief is a frustrating odyssey of doctor-hopping and taking overlapping medications; and after all is said and done, their pain remains. Many simply give up on the idea of finding relief. But living with chronic pain need not guarantee a miserable existence. Your life can be better—perhaps much better—if you understand your options and you are willing to pursue the physical, emotional, and spiritual changes that will reduce your pain and give you more control over it.

What can you do to ensure that your treatment has the best possible outcome? How can you manage your care, your body, your mind, and the logistics of your life to maximize your ability to live life to the fullest? Your best hope for minimized pain and a return to a normal life is a comprehensive strategy that counteracts the emotional, physical, and spiritual limitations of pain. Learning new ways of doing ordinary tasks and different ways of thinking about pain may reduce the medication you need and may even eliminate your need for it, so that you can not only live with chronic pain but live well. Some days are bound to be better than others, and the cure for most chronic pain eludes us, but we have an arsenal of tools—medications, spinal pumps, neurostimulators, numbing injections, nerve blocks, physical and psychological therapies that set the body and mind to work against pain—that can help you establish a state of détente with your pain. When people are motivated to embrace these tools, they enjoy happier, more fulfilling lives.

You may feel that your quest for an improved life is hopeless; in this book, you will find that that need not be the case. *Confronting Chronic Pain* will give you a thorough understanding of what might be going wrong in your body and what help (both standard and newer approaches) is available, and it will introduce actions you can take to improve your chances for success. Within these pages, you will become acquainted with treatments and actions that together constitute a successful approach to pain management:

- Medications (chapter 3)
- Techniques for changing the way you think about pain (chapter 4)
- Behavioral changes and physical therapies (chapter 5)
- Complementary medicine and alternative treatments (chapter 6)

The book will also help you to understand and cope with three important areas of a painful life that are often overlooked:

- Suffering and spiritual dilemmas (chapter 7)
- Minimizing pain's negative effects on your family (chapter 8)
- Becoming a patient in control (chapter 9)

No matter what the source of your discomfort or how long you have had it, chronic pain need not limit your capacity to live well. You can be helped and you can get better. No physician can give you a magic pill that will instantly and forever erase your pain. That does not exist. Nor is there a one-size-fits-all solution. But a multidisciplinary team of health care professionals who specialize in pain management will get you back on the road to a life that is not overshadowed or controlled by pain.

If you take away one important message after reading this book, let it be this: Never give up and never lose hope. Although life with unrelenting pain can be difficult, with the right tools you can cope and thrive, even when pain remains a part of your life.

Confronting Chronic Pain

The Science of Pain

Pain.

It is something we don't think about until we have it, and we are thankful when it goes away. But what if it does not? What if it remains and is always present to some degree?

Since we humans have populated the earth, physical pain has been a part of our existence. As the body's early warning system in response to imminent physical threat, it prompts us to guard our bodies. It immobilizes us after injury so that we have an opportunity to heal. Although pain is unwanted and unappreciated, our lives would be a good deal shorter without it, because we would not learn to move out of harm's way or seek treatment when faced with severe or life-threatening injuries. Imagine the consequences of keeping your hand in a flame or walking on a broken leg if pain didn't stop you. That is why individuals who have a rare inherited nerve disorder called *congenital analgesia* have reduced life expectancy. They cannot experience pain and are therefore unaware of injury or painful early symptoms of illness.

Pain Is Not All the Same

We all experience pain throughout our lives. We develop infections, sprain muscles, break bones, give birth. While this *acute pain* hurts, it is a healthy protective response that is usually temporary. It responds well to medication and dissipates as wounds heal, bones mend, and the body recuperates. When you develop a toothache, a dentist fills the cavity or

Most acute pain disappears on its own, yet pain that is untreated or treated inadequately can evolve into chronic pain. That is why aggressive postoperative pain management is wise, not only for a patient's comfort but also to curtail pain before it escalates.

performs a root canal. When you break your arm, a doctor sets the bone. In both instances, a medical professional identifies the underlying cause of your acute discomfort and prescribes treatment that usually eliminates the pain, and you get on with your life.

Chronic pain is a horse of a very different color (table 1.1). Unlike acute pain, it serves no protective purpose. If acute pain is Dr. Jekyll, then chronic pain is Mr. Hyde. It is the body's alarm system gone amok. Stuck in the "on" position for no discernible reason, chronic pain keeps sending pain signals after your illness retreats or your injury heals. Unlike acute pain, chronic pain often manifests in ways that are not easily observed or treated, appearing suddenly without warning and seemingly without cause. Regardless of the source, chronic pain is more than a symptom. It is a disease unto itself, pain that sometimes gets better or

TABLE 1.1 Comparing acute and chronic pain

Acute pain	Chronic pain
Warns of imminent bodily harm	Serves no useful purpose
A symptom of illness, injury, or surgery	A disease
Well understood by health care professionals	Misunderstood by most health care professionals
Easily diagnosed	Can be difficult to diagnose
Easily treated in the short term	May require long-term or indefinite treatment
Usually treated by a primary physician	May require treatment strategy that is coordinated by a pain specialist
Typically resolved with medication	Often requires multifaceted treatment
Rarely affects psychological or social health	Can cause anxiety, depression, insomnia, feelings of alienation, and other psychological problems
Does not affect spiritual health	Often triggers spiritual crises
Does not affect long-term quality of life	Often diminishes long-term functionality and well-being

worse but may never disappear entirely. Many otherwise healthy people who live with chronic pain are disabled for weeks, months, or the remainder of their lives if they are not successfully treated.

Categorizing Pain

Treatment for an acute illness or injury is predicated on the source of the problem. We reset broken bones, prescribe antibiotics for bacterial infections, and stitch wounds closed. Deciding on the right type of treatment for chronic pain is more difficult, because identifying its origin can be challenging, and often it is impossible. In some cases, a complete cure may not be possible even when the underlying condition is discovered.

Appropriate treatment depends on the type of pain experienced. *Nociceptive pain* is acute pain that usually responds well to medication. With the exception of arthritis, this type of pain is usually time limited—it stops when tissue heals and *nociceptors,* special nerve endings that react to potentially damaging stimuli, no longer detect impending injury or damage. Our bodies have millions of pain-sensing nociceptors, with the highest concentrations in the head, the mouth, the hands, and the feet. (Fewer nociceptors are found in the internal organs, which are more protected and less prone to injury.) Nociceptive pain may be *somatic* (it stems from damaged skin, bones, or muscles) or *visceral* (it occurs in the stomach, intestines, or other internal organs). Somatic pain can be a sharp, dull, aching, or throbbing sensation concentrated in a single location. Activity aggravates somatic pain, while rest improves it. Visceral pain is activated by nociceptors in the chest, the abdomen, or the pelvis. It tends to wax and wane, and the sensation is more diffuse, making it difficult to pinpoint.

Neuropathic pain is produced by an injury or a malfunction in the nervous system. Compared to nociceptive pain, neuropathy is more likely to be chronic, and it may persist for months or years after the damaged tissues heal. A neuropathic pain signal no longer represents an alarm about ongoing or impending injury; it is the alarm system itself that malfunctions, sending continuous stimulation that the brain perceives as pain. Patients with this type of pain often describe it as stabbing, burning, shooting, tingling, or like an electric shock that radiates beyond its point of origin. Shingles, diabetic neuropathy, fibromyalgia, and complex regional pain syndrome are common causes of neuropathic pain; some components of cancer pain are also neuropathic. Nerves that are inflamed, infiltrated, compressed by tumors, or strangulated by scar tissue may also become chronically painful. Not surprisingly, neuropathic pain is more difficult to treat than acute pain. It responds less well to *analgesics* (pain-relieving drugs) and other conventional pain treatments. Because neuropathic pain results from a damaged nervous system, it cannot always be reversed, but it may improve with medication and other treatments. Some chronic pain results from a complex mix of nociceptive and neuropathic factors (table 1.2).

Although persistent pain is a widespread problem, it remains something of an anomaly that is subject to misunderstandings and myths.

TABLE 1.2   Examples of nociceptive, neuropathic, and combined pain

Nociceptive pain conditions	Neuropathic pain conditions	Conditions with nociceptive and neuropathic pain
A cut or bruise	Carpal tunnel syndrome	Fibromyalgia
Broken bones	Migraine headaches	Myofascial pain
Osteoarthritis	Diabetic neuropathy	Cancer pain
Osteoporosis	Herpes zoster (shingles)	
Rheumatoid arthritis	Complex regional pain syndrome	
Postoperative pain	Phantom-limb pain	
	Chemotherapy-induced neuropathy	
	Pain from multiple sclerosis, stroke, or Parkinson's disease	

Here are six common myths about chronic pain:

1. Chronic pain cannot be cured. You just have to live with it.
   Although chronic pain cannot always be eliminated, treatment alternatives can help to reduce and control it.
2. Complaining about pain or seeking treatment is a sign of weakness.
   Pain is a very real problem. It can devastate physical, social, psychological, and spiritual well-being, but it can also be greatly improved with various therapies. Seeking treatment is an important step in the quest to live a better life.
3. When medical tests find no cause for pain, the source is usually psychological.
   Chronic pain is a complex medical issue that often defies standard diagnostic tools. Pinpointing the exact causes can be difficult and is not always possible.
4. Ignoring pain makes it disappear.
   Usually the opposite is true. Ignored chronic pain not only does not go away; it frequently becomes worse.
5. People can learn to work through their pain.
   Everyone who has pain has limits. Exceeding those limits can make pain worse.
6. Treating chronic pain requires long-term pain medication that leads to drug addiction.
   Many painkilling drugs, especially opioids, can safely treat chronic pain. Not all people with chronic pain need opioids; most who do need them do not become addicted.

The Ouch Response: The Mechanics of Pain

Throughout history, humans have debated the exact source of pain. Ancient tribes credited spirits and evil influences as the cause. Egyptians believed pain radiated from the heart. The early Greeks were the first to correctly understand that the brain and the nervous system produce the perception of pain and that pain is an emotion rather than a physical sensation. Not until 1,800 years later was a supporting hypothesis for this theory developed, when Leonardo da Vinci and other astute Renaissance thinkers correctly suspected that the brain is the body's control center for sensation and receives messages from the spinal cord. Da Vinci wrote, "The deeper the feeling, the greater the pain." Yet, as recently as the 1970s, we were still in the dark about pain and how the brain influences what we feel when we hurt. Pain was seen as a naturally occurring by-product of an underlying condition that people needed to suffer as a normal part of life. Four decades later, we know that approach was primitive and harmful. We now recognize chronic pain as real, even though it cannot be measured or seen on a scanning test and cannot always be explained.

Pain occurs within a fraction of a second after cutting a finger or breaking a bone. The immediate pain you feel is actually the result of a sophisticated bodily response of the *central nervous system* (the brain and the spinal cord) and the *peripheral nervous system* (the network of sensory nerve fibers in skin, muscles, and bones that feed information to the spinal cord and the brain). Your nervous systems coordinate voluntary functions (walking, talking, chewing) and regulate involuntary movements (breathing, heart rate, blood pressure). In a nutshell, when damage or injury occurs, sensory nerves send impulses to the spinal cord, which then forwards the signals on to areas of the brain that control sensation (you feel the pain) and emotional response (you react to it). Sounds simple, but even though the pain process is immediate, it is quite elaborate. A more thorough explanation begins at the source of pain: the nerves.

Pathways to and from the Brain

When nociceptors detect harmful stimuli, they send an electrical impulse to a part of the spinal cord called the *dorsal horn,* the spine's relay station for incoming and outgoing sensations. Nerve cells in the spine determine which impulses receive priority: sharp or severe pain signals travel instantly to the brain, while moderate signals advance more slowly. Weak pain messages, the type that occur with a bruise or a shallow cut, may not advance to the brain at all.

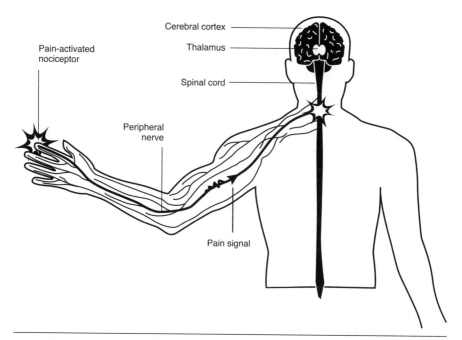

Cerebral cortex

Thalamus

Pain-activated
nociceptor

Spinal cord

Peripheral
nerve

Pain signal

FIGURE 1.1. Nociceptive impulses travel along peripheral nerves to the spinal cord and on to the brain.

Pain signals travel along the *ascending pathway* from the spine to the brain (figure 1.1). When the brain has processed these messages, it sends an appropriate response back down the *descending pathway* to the point of origin. Nonpainful sensations, such as touch and temperature, use a different pathway. Pain is so critical to survival that the central nervous system has its own backup system; if one pathway is damaged, another processes pain signals. Even though we all have these same pathways, our memories, thoughts, and emotions affect sensations sent from the brain, producing individual differences in our perception of pain.

The Gate-Control Theory

From the time of the ancient Greeks, pain was believed to be a simple process that traveled a straightforward pathway from damaged or inflamed tissue directly to the brain. In 1644, French philosopher René Descartes included a drawing in *Treatise of Man* illustrating his idea of how pain navigates through the body. The artwork of a boy with his foot in a fire shows the painful "disturbance" moving from the foot through the spinal cord and into the brain. Descartes wrote that painful sensations worked in the same way as "by pulling on one end of a rope one makes to strike at the same instant a bell which hangs at the end." His simplistic idea held until 1965, when scientists Ronald Melzack and Patrick Wall proposed a different hypothesis known as the Gate-Control Theory. They suggested that pain pathways are regulated by nerve cells in the spinal cord that act as biological "gates," opening to let pain through or closing to stop it. For the first time, scientists had a neurobiological basis to study and further understand pain. Melzack and Wall established at least a superficial understanding of what happens when chronic pain occurs: the gates get stuck in the open position and rogue pain signals travel unchecked to the brain.

The concept that pain is diminished or eliminated when the gates are closed was a revelation for scientists and a boon for patients. It profoundly changed pain treatment and initiated the field of pain management as a medical specialty. We now have many methods of closing the gates to curtail painful sensation, including medications and other treatments that target the body and the mind. Acupuncture, applying heat or cold, and other therapies initiate competing sensations that interrupt nerve impulses on the ascending pathway to the brain. Other treatments block disruptive signals. Massaging an aching muscle is one example. Applying pressure sends a competing signal that prevents pain signals from getting through the gate and reaching the brain; the result is diminished pain. The brain, with its complex stew of emotions, memories, expectations, and other psychological factors, is capable of dual roles: it can be pain's closest ally or its strongest adversary. What we think affects how we process pain signals; our thoughts can hold the gates open or swing them closed.

Why Ignoring Pain Makes It Worse

In addition to its persistent nature, chronic pain differs from acute pain in another significant and detrimental way: it is self-perpetuating. The body's pain system is adaptable and can react negatively to the duress of long-term pain. When nerve cells in the spinal cord and the brain form memories of resistant pain, they tend to respond to new stimuli, even less painful stimuli, in the same way. This is the phenomenon of *central sensitization,* when overexcited neurons exaggerate sensitivity to pain. People with shingles, for example, often report that the touch of the lightest clothing or bedsheet feels like terrible

burning. These pain-induced changes to the nervous system are long-lasting. Chronic pain may continue even when the original cause is eliminated. This fact underscores the importance of breaking the cycle of pain while the nervous system still has the ability to do so.

Chronic pain also erodes functionality and cognitive ability. *Positron emission tomography* (PET) scans—noninvasive diagnostic tests that produce three-dimensional images of the brain's metabolic activity—of people with chronic back pain show that areas of the brain that are normally at rest remain active when chronic pain is present. This ever-present brain activity causes fatigue, depression, forgetfulness, reduced concentration, and other cognitive problems.[1]

Passing the Pain Baton

The body's sensory pathways are paved with billions of *neurons,* nerve cells that shuttle signals between the body and the brain. Neurons (table 1.3) communicate with each other by releasing chemical messages called *neurotransmitters.* The brain releases different neurotransmitters to modulate sleep and mood, direct your heart to beat and your lungs to breathe, and regulate numerous bodily processes. Pain signals move from nerve to nerve in the same way. Once released by a neuron, a neurotransmitter travels across the *synapse* (the space between nerve cells) to *receptors* on the surface of the neighboring neuron (figure 1.2). (Neurons have countless receptors; each one is a unique lock-and-key mechanism that is activated by temperature, touch, movement, or a specific chemical message.) Some neurotransmitters act like brakes and inhibit pain messages, while others excite the receiving neuron to initiate an electrical impulse

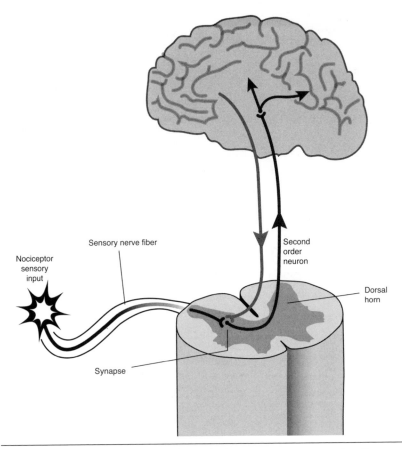

FIGURE 1.2. Neurons relay pain impulses and other sensory messages primarily through chemical synapses. Certain nonpainful stimuli (rubbing, touch, pressure, exercise, physical therapy, mind-body therapies, etc.) that enter the same synapse can close pain gates and inhibit pain signals from passing on to the next neuron ("second order neuron"), which carries the message up to the brain.

that travels the length of the nerve and then triggers the release of its own neurotransmitters at the far end of the nerve, repeating the synapse-spanning process from neuron to neuron until the message reaches the brain. The process works much like a relay race: one runner passes a baton to another runner, who either drops the baton (the nerve does not fire in response to the neurotransmitter) or receives it and carries it forward to the next runner (the nerve fires and sends the neurotransmitter across the synapse to the next neuron). Multiple neurotransmitters may

TABLE 1.3   The role of neurons in the body

Neuron types	Activity
Autonomic neurons	Coordinate involuntary automatic bodily functions
Brain neurons	Facilitate behavior, thought, and bodily functions
Spinal neurons	Conduct impulses to and from the brain
Motor neurons	Activate muscles and organs
Sensory neurons	Interface with the physical world

simultaneously enter a synapse, influencing the reaction of the receiving neuron.

Substance P

When tissue becomes inflamed or damaged, the nerves from that area release *substance P* ("P" for pain) signaling the nervous system that this area hurts. Some evidence shows that substance P also suppresses the immune system and reduces the body's supply of natural painkillers. Levels of substance P have been found to be significantly higher in people with rheumatoid arthritis or fibromyalgia.[2] The discovery of substance P, which is also involved in muscle contraction, salivary secretion, and the vomiting reflex, was an important piece of the pain puzzle. Future studies and a greater understanding of this pain messenger may lead to development of new analgesics that inhibit the nervous system's production of substance P.

Other neurotransmitters also influence pain. *Glutamate,* one of the brain's most powerful and abundant chemicals, stimulates memory, learning, and other vital functions. It may also be a key chemical involved in pain signals. Ordinarily, the brain maintains a delicate balance of glutamate, controlling the amount released and quickly clearing it from receptors. Insufficient glutamate levels can cause psychosis and coma, while an overabundance literally excites cells to death. Gamma-amino butyric acid prevents nerve cells from firing and may be part of natural processes that diminish or limit the sensation of pain. *Serotonin* and *norepinephrine* decrease pain signals, especially in combination. Bal-

SENSORY RECEPTORS PRODUCE DIFFERENT SENSATIONS

Nociceptors are just one of the body's sensory input mechanisms.

- Thermoreceptors sense heat, cold, and temperature changes.
- Mechanoreceptors are responsible for touch, pressure, sounds, and motion (including equilibrium).
- Direct chemoreceptors detect taste and changes in oxygen levels.
- Distant chemoreceptors make smell possible.
- Photoreceptors respond to light and enable vision.

anced amounts of serotonin stabilize mood and help to prevent nerves in the brain from firing excessively. Antidepressants that enhance serotonin and norepinephrine can be effective tools to reduce neuropathic pain.

Endorphins

Pain impulses entering the brain trigger the release of *endorphins* into the blood system. Endorphins are the body's own happy pills. They create the rush of pleasurable feelings we experience from meditation, laughter, eating chocolate or chili peppers, and sex. A body under extreme stress releases massive quantities of endorphins to reduce the perception of pain signals that reach the brain, enhancing immune system response and lowering stress in the process. Endorphins work like a more robust version of morphine, replacing pain with calmness and euphoria. They create the "runner's high" brought about by intense aerobic activity. This endorphin high partially explains how combat soldiers can fight on after they have been badly wounded—pain messages are likely subdued by endorphins flooding the nervous system, along with other inhibitory signals from the brain that close the spinal pain gates. Both phenomena illustrate an invaluable lesson for anyone with chronic pain: when you are highly motivated to improve your condition, you are better positioned to manage your pain and get more out of life. Deliberately raising endorphin levels with physical activity, behavioral changes, and targeted thinking can modulate and reduce chronic pain.

The Placebo-Endorphin Connection

A *placebo* is fake medication. It is the so-called control in clinical trials that determines whether observed treatment differences are due to real medication or to a patient's belief that the substance she was given will improve her condition. It is a mistake to assume that individuals who respond to a placebo do not have a legitimate medical condition or true pain. A considerable body of research shows that the mind-body process that engages the brain's self-healing mechanisms is at work. In the case of chronic pain, experts speculate that the anticipation of a beneficial reaction provokes the release of endorphins, creating a sense of well-being. Not so long ago, explaining the placebo effect as a physiological process that might have a place alongside "real" medicine would have been thought preposterous. The discovery of endorphins, however, offered a clearer picture of how these neurotransmitters affect pain perception and how they can be manipulated by medication, placebo, meditation, and other mind-body therapies.

A classic study in the late 1970s demonstrated the neurochemical response of placebos. Among patients who had dental surgery, some were given intravenous (IV) drips of morphine, while others received only saline. As expected, some patients in the placebo (saline) group reported improved pain levels, while others did not. Then the researchers added naloxone to the IV drips of the placebo group. Naloxone—a drug used to treat overdoses of heroin and morphine—counteracts endorphins by blocking opioid receptors. The researchers suspected if the placebo had worked by engaging endorphins, naloxone would negate its benefit. In fact, that is what happened. Patients who had experienced diminished pain from the placebo effect now felt sharply increased pain. The study showed that the placebo effect—an action of the mind—dulls pain by the same biochemical route as opioids.[3] A more recent study suggested that conditioning might also invoke the placebo response. Mice that were given morphine or aspirin before being subjected to pain responded similarly when they were subjected to pain again, even when the medication was withheld.[4]

Contrary to earlier thinking, experiencing a positive reaction from a placebo does not mean that the responder is weak-willed or suggestible or that his underlying problem is psychological. It does mean that he has used his mind, either consciously or subconsciously, to engage his body's healing apparatus. Patients who expect that their pain will be reduced create from their minds the very neurophysiology that brings about that result. To the patient, it does not matter whether the improvement is physiological or psychological; he simply feels better. Whether the beneficial nature of a treatment is real or imagined isn't the most important question. A more significant issue is what the placebo effect demonstrates: that your mind can greatly influence your body and your health, including chronic pain, down to the smallest cell.

If the placebo works so well in trials, why not use it therapeutically? That is a much-discussed and controversial issue among members of the medical community. Some doctors argue that prescribing "fake" treatment is not only deceptive but immoral and unethical as well, because doing so withholds beneficial medication from patients in need and ignores the concept of informed consent. At least one study, however, shows that a placebo appears to work even when patients know the substance they are taking has no medicinal properties. Researchers at Harvard Medical School tested this theory of "placebo without deception." They randomly assigned a group of 80 patients with irritable bowel syndrome (IBS) to two groups. One group was told that they were being given "placebo pills made of an inert substance, like sugar pills, that have been shown in clinical studies to produce significant improvement in IBS symptoms through mind-body self-healing processes," and they were given pill bottles that were clearly labeled "placebo." The control group received no medication or placebo. After three weeks, nearly twice as many patients in the placebo group reported relief from their symptoms as patients in the control group.[5]

Another argument against routine use of placebos is that people do not all respond to the suggestion of healing in the same way; biological, psychosocial, and even genetic factors may influence a person's reaction. Some health care professionals sharply disagree, citing medical literature that shows positive outcomes in 30 to 90 percent of patients who receive a placebo. Although we know that certain individuals are more susceptible to placebos than others, this finding suggests that many people might benefit from a placebo and be free of side effects and the risk of medications.

The Brain Takes Over

For the past 300 years, our understanding of pain has been dominated by the idea that the human body is a complex machine that is separate from the process of perception. Pain, however, is a subjective experience that cannot be divided from an individual's mental state, memories, environment, and mind-set. These factors can be so influential that they cause the brain to either elicit or abolish the experience of pain, independently of what is occurring elsewhere in the body.

Even though you are conscious of pain as soon as you experience a cut or a broken bone, the sensation occurs only after the neural signal has passed from the site of the injury, through the spinal cord, to the brain. The brain has no single pain center. Collective input from different areas of the brain determines your response. Pain signals sent to the brain are first received in the *thalamus,* an important message relay center between the brain and the body. The thalamus then forwards the signals to the *cerebral cortex,* where thought occurs. This part of the brain is the mechanism that identifies the location of the injury and assesses the severity of the damage. It also determines how the body should react, directing blood and nutrients to the site of the injury, sending pain-reducing endorphins into the bloodstream, and initiating pain-reduction messages that travel down the descending pathways.

As pain messages are processed by the cerebral cortex, they are simultaneously received in the *limbic system,* a portion of the brain involved in memory and emotional response. There, your past pain experiences, current mood, and all other activities going on in your nervous system are tossed into the mix. Pain signals produce a memory of past experiences that helps the brain to categorize and identify the stimulus. Messages arriving in the limbic system generate immediate thoughts ("Uh oh, this is serious") and emotions ("I'm hurt!" or "I'm fine"). The stronger the response from the limbic system, the more intensely you feel pain. (If you cry from certain types of pain but not others, the limbic system is responsible.) Oddly, the brain has no nociceptors and does not directly sense pain. In fact, most brain surgery is performed with only a local anesthetic for the scalp and the skull.

The value you assign to pain has extraordinary influence on how you feel it. Pain viewed with stress, depression, or anxiety is felt more strongly than pain experienced when you are hopeful, upbeat, or encouraged. If you were fired from your job just before you hit your thumb with a hammer, you would probably react in a very different way than if you were on your honeymoon or if you received a pay raise just before the mishap occurred. Past experience also plays a role. You would probably recover more quickly from that hammer injury if you had the same experience before and suffered no adverse consequences. If a previous episode with the hammer sent you to the hospital for stitches, your thumb then became infected, and you needed antibiotics, you might feel more pain the next time you hit your thumb in exactly the same way.

The Perception of Pain

It is surprisingly difficult to clinically assess pain, because each of us experiences it differently. On a numerical scale, where zero is no pain at all and 10 is unbearable, one person's 4 may be another person's 9, even though the pain is exactly the same. Pain is whatever the patient says it

TABLE 1.4   Factors that influence pain perception

Factor	How it affects the perception of pain
Gender	Women are more sensitive than men to pain
Age	Growing older may decrease sensitivity to pain or an individual's reaction to it
Fatigue	An unrested body feels more pain
Stress or anxiety	Both emotions increase pain perception
Mood	Depression and other emotional disturbances can increase pain.
Memory	Past experiences with pain can influence perception of future pain. Your belief in your doctor or in your own ability to cope can make pain better.

is. This subjectivity, along with other physiological and psychological factors that influence perception (table 1.4), is part of what makes treatment of chronic pain so difficult.

Pain in Special Populations

Women

Historically, much of the pain reported by women was assumed to be a figment of their imagination, a result of being overemotional, oversensitive, or weak. Several studies, in fact, show that many physicians still downplay women's complaints of pain and prescribe less aggressive treatment than they do for men with the same symptoms. Presented with a man and a woman who describe the same chronic pain, physicians are more likely to prescribe painkillers for the man and only sedatives for the woman.[6]

Women more often have chronic pain than men, and when they do, it tends to be more intense and longer-lasting. Women suffer more frequently from headaches, autoimmune disorders, fibromyalgia, rheumatoid arthritis, and irritable bowel syndrome. Researchers aren't sure why this is, but several studies point to perceptions of pain, genetics, and variable psychological factors between genders. Some experts believe that male and female pain systems behave differently, possibly because women have more nerve receptors and are more strongly influenced by estrogen and other hormones.[7] Studies support the notion that estrogen acts as a pain switch and that menstrual cramps may alter brain micro-structures in a manner similar to the way chronic pain does. In laboratory experiments, when female mice were deprived of estrogen, they developed higher pain thresholds, similar to those of the male mice.[8] Women also tend to seek treatment for pain sooner than men and recover more quickly. They are more likely to try different coping skills and are less likely to allow pain to control their lives.

Older Adults

According to the National Institutes of Health, about half of older Americans who live alone have chronic pain. As we age, we become more vulnerable to chronic pain and conditions that cause it. The wear and tear of decades takes its toll, muscles atrophy, joints weaken, activity levels decrease, and we are more susceptible to arthritis, cancer, osteoporosis, and other debilitating disorders. Falls and accidents are more likely to occur, and we recover more slowly than youthful individuals. Many people in this age category are socially detached; this condition provides fertile ground for developing anxiety disorders that intensify painful symptoms. Older people, however, complain about pain less often. Many elderly people consider pain to be an inevitable part of aging and therefore do not seek clinical help. Nevertheless, pain is the number one complaint of older Americans; one in five regularly takes painkilling medication.[9]

Because older people are often reticent to discuss their pain or find it difficult to describe, diagnosis and treatment can be difficult. Pain medications may also be problematic. Seniors may fear strong analgesics or experience especially adverse reactions. They are also more likely to take multiple medications for high blood pressure, cholesterol, or other health issues, which can interact negatively with analgesics. Many older adults may forgo pain medicines altogether because they cannot afford the cost.

Military Veterans

Traumatic physical, psychological, or sexual events can create chronic pain. Experiencing the horrors of war certainly qualifies as traumatic, and many soldiers return home with wounds, but not all injuries are visible. An estimated 68 percent of veterans of the Iraq conflict have post-traumatic stress disorder (PTSD). Many more—81 percent—have chronic pain (about the same percentage as for Vietnam vets).[10] Either PTSD or chronic pain can wreak havoc on an individual's life. When people have both disorders, as many vets do, the adverse life impact—anxiety, depression, anger, fear, and panic—is more intense than if they had only one or the other. Effective treatment needs to address both issues.

Treating combat injuries has always been a challenge for the medical community. Each new conflict seems to introduce injuries that require more innovative and sophisticated therapies. That has certainly been the case with modern wars in the Middle East. Although the use of body armor and improved treatment on the battlefield saves the lives of thousands of soldiers, many who return home suffer from chronic pain. According to data from the Department of Defense, military physicians wrote nearly 3.8 million prescriptions for pain medication in 2009, more than quadruple the number of such prescriptions in 2001. One in five soldiers who returns to the United States with deployment-related concussions has chronic headaches 15 or more days a month, a rate that is almost five times as high as the general population's rate.[11]

Underrepresented Populations

While the chronic pain experience in America is not ideal for most people, a combination of problems magnifies the issue for poor and minority populations, making them particularly vulnerable. Fifty million Americans, many of them people of color, have no health care insurance, so pain treatment is beyond their reach (it remains to be seen whether health care reform will eliminate the problem). Cultural and linguistic barriers often keep many people in these populations from seeking treatment. Some view pain fatalistically, considering it an unpreventable fate. Many rely on unconventional treatments as a first line of defense for pain management, seeing a doctor only when their pain becomes intolerable. They may equate being a good patient with not complaining. Others consider asking for help to be a sign of weakness.

Racial and ethnic groups cope with pain in significantly different ways.

Some people in various groups may not recognize when pain becomes serious or chronic, or they fear the addictive potential of strong drugs. Often, when members of minority populations do seek medical assistance, the pain assessment, diagnosis, and prescribed treatment they receive are inadequate. People of color have less access to pain-management services than other populations and are less likely to receive pain medication; studies in various states show that pharmacies in low-income and predominantly nonwhite neighborhoods do not maintain sufficient stocks of opioid medications to treat chronic pain.

SUMMARY POINTS
- Pain is a complex and elaborate process that involves both body and mind.
- Chronic pain is different from acute pain and requires a different treatment approach.
- The source of chronic pain can be difficult to identify and sometimes remains a mystery.
- Left untreated, chronic pain can intensify the body's response to pain.

Chronically Painful Conditions

Although the causes of chronic pain cannot always be identified, an underlying health condition is often the culprit. Persistent pain may result from arthritis, back pain, headaches, or other chronic disorders and diseases that do not resolve from treatment. Your doctor may order a variety of diagnostic procedures to rule out specific disorders in an effort to identify the source of your pain.

Arthritis

More than 100 types of *arthritis* can affect the joints. Arthritis develops when the joints become inflamed or when the protective cartilage that normally functions as a shock absorber between bones roughens and becomes thin. Without the padding of healthy, slick cartilage, joint movement becomes painful. Arthritic joints may look or feel larger than normal, and they may feel stiff, warm, or tender to the touch. Moving the joint can cause discomfort ranging from mildly uncomfortable to very painful, limiting flexibility and range of motion and in some cases producing a crackling sound called *crepitation*. When joints become inflamed and the bone ends become thicker, *bone spurs,* painful bumpy growths of new bone, may develop. Most arthritis is chronic. It often responds to the right kind of medication and lifestyle changes, but it cannot be cured.

Osteoarthritis

The most prevalent type of arthritis is *osteoarthritis* (OA), chronic joint degeneration that forms when cartilage deteriorates from age. Also referred to as "degenerative joint disease," OA occurs equally in men and women before age 55, but it is more common in women after that age. OA can be hereditary; if one or both of your parents have it, you are more likely to get it as well. It may develop sooner if you have had a fracture or other traumatic injury affecting the joint. Osteoarthritis also results from repetitive joint stress. Jobs that require squatting, kneeling, lifting, or climbing throughout the day may cause this type of damage over time. Premature OA is common among quarterbacks, baseball pitchers, and others who routinely subject their joints to inordinate load and stress. Even technology can be problematic. "Blackberry thumb" and "cell phone elbow" develop from prolonged cell phone use that stresses thumbs and elbows more than they are designed to withstand. Left untreated, both conditions can develop into tendonitis or chronically painful OA. People who play video games for hours each day may sustain similar injuries.

For most people, the characteristic early-stage aching of OA is easily treated. It can progressively worsen, however, until it limits even minimal movement, so getting adequate treatment early on and learning how to manage symptoms make a noticeable difference. Treatment begins with a visit to your primary care doctor and ordinarily involves *nonsteroidal anti-inflammatory drugs* (NSAIDs) to reduce pain and inflammation. These medications are effective, but they can cause gastrointestinal problems and increase blood pressure, so they are not ideal for the long term. Aside from medication, acupuncture and applications of cold or heat (or alternately applying both) can help. Some people find that *capsaicin* skin cream (Zostrix) temporarily relieves painful joints. (Capsaicin is the heat-producing ingredient in chili peppers.) Advanced cases require consultation with a *rheumatologist,* a physician who specializes in the treatment of arthritis.

Being overweight contributes to osteoarthritis, as it places abnormal stress on knees, ankles, and hips. Shedding even a few pounds can lessen pressure on weight-bearing joints and decrease pain. Exercising may seem impossible if you suffer from painful arthritis, but that is precisely what can improve your condition. Your physician or a physical therapist can recommend low-impact exercises to strengthen the supporting muscles around your joints so that you gradually build flexibility and increase your range of motion (swimming pool exercises are especially easy on the joints). Massage therapy by a practitioner who is experienced with joint pain may also help. Learning to bend, walk, sit, and move in a way that protects joints and causes less pain is also beneficial. Severe arthritis pain can be relieved for several weeks to several months by injecting a *corticosteroid* (a synthetic anti-inflammatory hormone) or artificial joint fluid directly into the joint. When extreme pain persists despite all other treatments, surgical repair or a partial or total replacement of the joint may be recommended.

Nutritional supplements, especially glucosamine and chondroitin sulfate, are widely marketed as "natural" arthritis pain relievers. But do they work? Multiple studies have examined the effectiveness of these dietary supplements, with mixed results. The most comprehensive analysis, the Glucosamine/Chondroitin Arthritis Intervention Trial (GAIT) involved 1,583 patients age 40 or older with OA of the knee. In this research, glucosamine or chondroitin taken alone did not relieve pain more effectively than a placebo. Taken in combination, however, glucosamine and chondroitin were somewhat effective for moderate to severe pain; they did not benefit those with mild pain.[1] (These results need to be confirmed by further research, because the moderate-to-severe pain group was small.) A few small studies have shown that glucosamine slows the progression of arthritis, but other studies, including the secondary phase of GAIT research, did not. Until more definitive information is available, talk to your physician about taking glucosamine and chondroitin for your arthritis. If you decide to try these supplements, remember that they are not regulated as drugs, so it is important to use a reputable brand.

Rheumatoid Arthritis

Rheumatoid arthritis (RA) is less common but more threatening than osteoarthritis, because it can lead to permanent disability. RA is an *autoimmune disease,* a disorder that develops when the immune system attacks healthy tissue for unknown reasons. In the case of RA, the immune system attacks the *synovium,* the thin membrane lining the joints. Opposing joints on both sides of the body are affected; if RA develops in your right elbow, it will probably show up in your left elbow as well. Like osteoarthritis, RA symptoms include joint inflammation and pain. But unlike osteoarthritis, which gradually worsens but improves with treatment, RA is systemic—it aggressively spreads throughout the body, destroying joints, tendons, ligaments, and bones. The result is extreme pain, fatigue, difficulty sleeping, and sometimes, shortness of breath. RA is more common among women, middle-aged folks, and smokers. People with RA may have intense bouts of pain alternating with long periods without symptoms. Others suffer from pain that never seems to fade and intensifies over time.

RA cannot be cured, but early treatment can curtail its progression. In some cases, it may respond to the same treatments used for osteoarthritis. Most NSAIDs, however, are not ideal for RA because of their long-term side effects. If you have RA, you should be treated by a rheumatologist, who will likely recommend a *disease-modifying antirheumatic drug* (DMARD) to suppress your immune system, decrease pain and swelling, and stop progressive joint damage. DMARD therapy should be started if an NSAID regimen does not produce a favorable response within three months; DMARDs are most successful against the progression of RA when they are started soon after diagnosis. Methotrexate is one of the most common and effective DMARDs used for RA. Combining it with another DMARD or prednisone (a steroid) often produces a better response. Most people with RA need to take medication for the rest of their lives.

Even though DMARDs offer life-altering improvements for many, we do not know enough about them to determine their long-term safety and effectiveness. Because they work by suppressing the immune system, they are not the right choice for all patients. Researchers are exploring ways to combine DMARDs with other medications and develop newer RA drugs with fewer serious side effects. Studies of one oral medication, fostamatinib disodium, taken with methotrexate or other similar medications, are ongoing to determine whether it blocks immune system cells that attack and destroy bone and cartilage. When joint damage is extreme and other treatments fail, *biologics* may be prescribed. Used alone or in combination with other medications, these genetically engineered proteins target only specific parts of the immune system that prompt RA, leaving the rest of the immune system unaffected. Biologics developed exclusively to treat RA (Enbrel, Rituxan, Humira, and others) appear to work well and carry fewer risks than other systemic therapies; however, they are a recent discovery and are not yet well studied. If biologics also fail to provide adequate relief, joint replacement surgery is a last resort.

Gout

Another type of arthritis affects a single joint, usually in the feet, and especially in the big toe. *Gout* develops when concentrations of uric acid, a by-product of naturally occurring *purines* in human and plant cells, accumulate in the blood and form small crystals in the joints. (Not everyone who has high levels of uric acid develops gout.) Historically, a purine-rich diet was believed to cause the "disease of kings." In fact, although diet may contribute to gout, an increased level of uric acid in the kidneys is more frequently the cause. Small crystals of uric acid—the same type that causes some kidney stones—create characteristic inflammation, stiffness, and pain in the joints. Risk factors include obesity, hypertension, and genetics. Gout is more common among people who take diuretic medications and those who have diabetes, kidney disease, anemia (including sickle-cell anemia), and blood cancers (including leukemia). Most people with gout are men over age 40. Women who develop gout ordinarily do so after menopause. We do not have a cure for gout, but it can be controlled with anti-inflammatory drugs, steroids, and other medicines that decrease uric acid in the blood. Effective gout medications reduce the need for a strict diet, but it is still important to understand how your diet can affect your symptoms, as you will see in chapter 5.

Cancer-Related Pain

Contrary to what most people believe, not everyone who has cancer suffers significant pain. Yet many of those with cancer do. Cancer pain is often undertreated, and too many people suffer needlessly. An analysis of 52 studies conducted over the past 40 years identified the prevalence of cancer pain: 64 to 80 percent of people with metastatic or advanced disease have pain, 59 percent of people undergoing treatment, and 33 percent of people who have completed treatment. More than one-third of people who have cancer describe their pain as moderate or severe.[2]

Cancer pain can be nociceptive (related to tissue damage) or neuropathic (from irritated or damaged nerves). Frequently it is a combination of both. Lasting pain may be caused by a tumor pressing on nerves, bones, or organs. It also develops when cancer destroys tissue, especially in people who have advanced disease. Chemotherapy is one of the most common ways to combat cancer, but it can cause many side effects, including chronic neuropathic pain in the extremities, bones, and joints. Many cancer-related neuropathies improve in time, but many do not. Radiation therapy less frequently causes the same type of pain that results from chemotherapy; but it sometimes relieves pain by reducing or destroying tumors that put painful pressure on tissues and nerves.

Treating cancer pain often requires high doses of opioids or therapies that are rarely used otherwise. Patients in severe pain may get relief from a pain pump implanted beneath the skin that delivers morphine or other potent medicines directly into the spinal fluid. Individuals with overwhelming cancer-related bone pain that does not respond to other treatments may benefit from *cementoplasty,* injections of special medical cement that strengthen and support the bone. Destroying rogue nerves may be the only way to deal with severe pain that does not respond to other treatments.

End-of-Life Pain

It is tragic that so many people spend their final months in terrible pain. It is also unnecessary. End-of-life pain is grossly undertreated in the United States. Many physicians are reluctant to administer powerful pain relievers that may also sedate patients and limit their ability to communicate effectively. People who are terminally ill and their loved ones often fear that stronger pain medicines will hasten death, yet research and clinical practice show that almost all pain at the end of a person's life can be managed in a way that relieves suffering and comforts the person without abbreviating life. End-of-life care that emphasizes minimization of pain is a growing medical specialty.

Fibromyalgia

Imagine profound widespread pain and overall stiffness that becomes worse with time and for which no cause can be found. You cannot get a decent night's sleep and you are always exhausted—getting out of bed seems to be beyond your capabilities. Any type of exertion is extremely painful. Headaches and nausea are commonplace. Your memory and cognitive abilities also suffer and you fall into a deep depression. Every day is a challenge, and your life falls apart. This is the nightmare of *fibromyalgia,* a disease that manifests no swelling, fever, or other telltale signs of illness. It is one of the most common chronic pain conditions, running in families and mostly affecting women between ages 20 and 40; yet we lack definitive diagnostic tests or treatment, and the cause remains a mystery. Some experts suspect bacterial or viral infections. Trauma, chronic sleep disturbance, emotional distress, and a variety of other factors seem to promote fibromyalgia in susceptible individuals. Some evidence suggests that it may be related to abnormal functioning of the *endocrine* (hormonal) *system* and incorrect signaling in regions of the brain that process pain.

For years, the medical community erroneously viewed fibromyalgia as a condition that people were imagining and were describing with overstated reports of pain. It is unclear whether this painful bedlam in the body *causes* other conditions or co-exists *with* them, but it is apparent that fibromyalgia pain is real. People with fibromyalgia are victimized by central sensitization; they suffer from exaggerated pain responses to sensory stimuli that are not ordinarily painful. Three well-respected studies found that people with fibromyalgia suffer from deficient levels of serotonin and norepinephrine combined with excessive amounts of pain-causing neurotransmitters, including substance P and glutamate.[3]

Characterized by tender and aching joints, muscles, and other soft tissues, fibromyalgia symptoms often overlap with indications of other chronically painful conditions. Neuropathic pain medicines, including pregabalin (Lyrica), duloxetine (Cymbalta), and milnacipran (Savella), usually improve fibromyalgia symptoms. Duloxetine and milnacipran also have an antidepressant effect. Other low-dose antidepressants help with sleep disturbance, fatigue, and depression. Anti-inflammatories and muscle relaxants address pain and stiffness, and some patients respond well to other medications, such as Amantadine, an antiviral medicine used to treat Parkinson's disease. Gradually building tolerance for exercise is critical for rehabilitation. Progress may be slow, because even the slightest activity can be exhausting and painful. Low-impact exercise, including aquatics and tai chi, builds strength and mobility while minimizing joint load. A regimen of gentle movement reduces pain and improves the person's quality of life and endurance.[4] Stress management and psychological therapies help overcome the debilitation and depression that many people who have fibromyalgia feel.

❁ FIBROMYALGIA

LISA WAS A 40-YEAR-OLD CORPORATE ATTORNEY who spent most of her time at her fast-paced, stressful job. Her problems began with low-back pain and pounding migraines that kept her at home on some days. Then other symptoms appeared: fatigue, flulike aching, sore muscles, and a general feeling of malaise. Lisa's condition continued to deteriorate until her symptoms more frequently kept her from work. Showering and dressing required unthinkable effort; even the slightest activity was out of the question. Her constant fight against pain left her exhausted, and she spent much of her time in bed. Lisa began to push friends and family away, which only made her feel more isolated with her pain. Alone and miserable, she could not shake her depression and the hopelessness of her future. She felt as though her body was betraying her. Lisa's primary physician diagnosed fibromyalgia and referred her to us.

We began with a complete physical exam and lab workup to eliminate other potential causes. Once we confirmed the diagnosis of fibromyalgia, we developed a comprehensive treatment plan that included medications to manage Lisa's headaches and muscle pain, an antidepressant to control her depression, and a sleeping aid to reduce her insomnia. Lisa also began physical therapy that included gentle stretching for a few minutes each day, progressing to 15-minute slow walks three times a week. Biweekly psychotherapy sessions were scheduled to help her cope with depression and other emotional issues that contributed to her suffering. As treatment progressed, Lisa began to sleep more soundly, and on most days, she felt less anxious and more confident in her ability to function. Her strength, stamina, and energy level continued to improve. As she slowly increased her exercise regimen, her symptoms receded until she felt about 50 percent better. Even though many tasks were still beyond her capability and she felt fatigued on some days, she could more frequently take care of herself and function fairly well. At this point, however, Lisa's improvement plateaued. Try as she might, she could not get any better. Much improved but no longer able to keep up with the demands of her career, she resigned her position and instead took on periodic freelance legal work. For Lisa, managing her symptoms would be a long-term effort. ○

Headaches

Everyone gets an occasional headache. We have a stressful day, spend too much time in front of computers, or struggle with family problems. While these head pains are annoying, they are ordinarily mild and temporary, disappearing on their own or after we pop a couple of over-the-counter pain relievers. Millions of people, however, suffer with frequent headaches that are so severe they cannot lift their heads or move without almost unbearable throbbing pain.

Effective treatment depends on the type of headache and a person's tolerance for side effects. When over-the-counter pain relievers fail to improve or eliminate headaches, prescription-strength medications can be taken as soon as symptoms develop. Short-acting pain medications that are intended to end a headache are referred to as abortive medications, whereas preventive drugs don't end headaches; rather, they reduce the frequency and strength of headaches. In all cases, practicing relaxation and stress reduction is necessary to minimize headaches and cope with them when they do occur. Avoiding certain triggering behaviors will also serve you well. Not everyone has the same *triggers,* so identifying what sets off your headaches is a first step in self-management. Many individuals find that maintaining a headache diary, like the examples shown at the website of the American Headache Society Committee for Headache Education (www.achenet.org/resources/headache _diaries), helps them to identify lifestyle behaviors that contribute to their headaches.

Caffeine, the world's most used drug, is a common trigger for many types of headaches, but it is also frequently added to analgesics to boost effectiveness. How can both facts be true? Caffeine is a stimulant. It activates pleasurable feelings in the same way cocaine does, revving up the nervous system and temporarily increasing alertness and energy. Regular caffeine intake also triggers dependence. If you routinely supply your body with caffeine, eliminating it abruptly can cause unpleasant effects, including headaches. This explains why you may wake up with a "weekend headache" when you sleep in and miss your regular morning cup of coffee—your body is in withdrawal. Your headache may disappear when you finally have your coffee, but it will probably return when the caffeine wears off. If morning coffee is your routine, it may even be possible to experience caffeine withdrawal headaches by the end of the day.

Researchers who reviewed the results of 57 headache studies found that half of all participants developed headaches as a result of caffeine withdrawal.[5] Gradually weaning yourself away from caffeine by substituting noncaffeine products (or skipping a cup here and there) will result in fewer withdrawal symptoms.

Cluster Headaches

Rare bouts of severe and quickly escalating headaches on one side of the head are called *cluster headaches.* A flurry of brief headaches may repeat during the day for a few weeks or several months, or resolve for months or years, only to reappear in the same pattern. Cluster headaches usually develop in men under age 30, particularly those who regularly drink alcohol and smoke. Treatment may include gradually tapered high doses of anti-inflammatory medication, breathing pure oxygen, and *triptans,* a type of medication that quickly stops some types of severe headaches.

Rebound Headaches

One of the most surprising facts about headaches is that they are often caused by the very medications we take to stop them. Over-the-counter pain relievers improve mild headache pain, but frequent use can make headaches worse. A cycle of pain is quickly established: the medications ease headaches for a while before wearing off. The pain returns, requiring even more medication. The key is to know how much to take and for how long—it is best not to exceed four doses per month. If your headaches persist, ask your doctor for a referral to a headache specialist or a neurologist for evaluation and treatment with preventive medications.

Treatment for *rebound headaches* begins by tapering off all short-acting headache and pain medicines, replacing them with low doses of long-acting analgesics, and minimizing use of abortive medications. Very low doses of methadone may be a better choice for many people who take Vicodin (a combination of the opioid hydrocodone bitartrate and acetaminophen), which is a narcotic for moderate to severe pain, for rebound headaches. As headaches become controlled, people should gradually taper off their use of long-acting pain medicines. A program of stress management and consistent routine can be enormously beneficial. Exercising, abstaining from cigarettes and other tobacco products, eating nutritionally balanced meals, and sleeping at about the same time every day can work wonders. It all takes discipline, but in a few months, persons who persevere are rewarded with dramatic improvement. Their headaches tend to be more infrequent and less painful, as they were before their rebound headaches began.

Migraines

"Like a hot knife piercing my skull." "Unimaginable pain I have never felt before." "An unending pounding in my head that does not stop." This is how people describe *migraine headaches*. More than just a headache, a migraine is a neurological disorder that affects the brain. Many sufferers are forced to spend days in a darkened room with eyes closed and minimal movement. Not all migraines are severe. Symptoms, frequency, and duration of migraines vary, but the result is often an intense pulsing or throbbing pain that can extend to the jaws, neck, and shoulders and may be accompanied by extreme sensitivity to light, sound, and movement (table 2.1). Individuals with chronic migraines frequently also develop superimposed rebound headaches from medication—they have both types of headaches simultaneously. In a common pattern, people begin having headaches when they are in their teens or twenties. As they con-

TABLE 2.1 Comparing ordinary headaches and migraines

Ordinary headache	Migraine
Occurs infrequently	Typically occurs 1 to 4 times per month
Mild aching or tension	Intensely painful pulsing or throbbing
Painful on top, front, or sides of the head	Usually painful on one side of the head
Pain limited to head	Pain also in the jaw, neck, or shoulders
Usually responds to over-the-counter medications	Usually requires stronger drugs and other therapies
Does not cause other symptoms	Often accompanied by dizziness, nausea, vomiting, and sensitivity to light, sound, and smell
Usually of short duration	May last for several hours or several days

tinue taking pain medication over the years, their headaches become more frequent and more painful. By the time most people with migraines see a pain specialist, they have already developed a pattern of frequent, even daily headaches.

There are four phases of a migraine:

1. Although they may not be aware of it, up to one-third of people experience subtle symptoms during the *premonitory* or *prodrome* phase that occurs a day or two before a migraine begins. These precursors may include a mood change, dizziness, gastrointestinal upset, or muscle stiffness. Some people notice that they develop unusual food cravings, yawn excessively, use the bathroom more or less than usual, or feel irritable or unusually tired. In some cases, rather than something specific, it is a vague feeling that something is just not right. Keeping a careful log of what you eat, drink, do, and feel will help you recognize premonitory symptoms (if you have them). Your log might reveal that you typically feel dizzy, have muscle stiffness, or crave chocolate on the night before you get a migraine. Recognizing these early warning symptoms may help you forestall a migraine if you then avoid your triggers, take good care of yourself, and, if needed, take preventive medication.

2. About one-third of people who have migraines experience *auras,* visual disturbances that appear 15 to 60 minutes before the pain begins. Auras may appear as flashes, stripes of light, blind spots, or squiggly lines in the vision. These are caused by waves of nerve dysfunction that ripple across the surface of the brain.

3. For many migraine sufferers, the headache phase is marked by moderate to severe throbbing pain that usually occurs on one side of the head but may be on both sides. This symptom may last for several hours or a few days. Some people also experience nausea, vomiting, and sensitivity to sound, light, odors, and movement.

4. The *postdrome* phase is the "migraine hangover," which may linger for a day or two after the headache ends. Fatigue, depression, and difficulty concentrating may occur during this phase.

Migraines run in families, and mounting evidence points to inherited vulnerability. They are a genetic disorder and usually result from a triggering event—they may not develop if you do not encounter a trigger that sets them off. The triggering event appears to cause neurons in the brain to release chemicals that excite nearby pain sensors and increase blood flow. (See "Migraine Triggers" at http://uhs.berkeley.edu/home/healthtopics/pdf/triggers.pdf.) Serotonin may be one chemical involved, since many migraine medications work by altering the way serotonin binds to receptors. Certain foods, low blood sugar, perfumes, fluctuating hormone levels before and during menstruation, and even changes in the weather are triggers in some people. Smoking and secondhand smoke narrow blood vessels in the brain and also act as migraine triggers. Skipping a meal or changing your sleep routine may be problematic if you are susceptible to migraines.

Triggers are cumulative. The more you have at one time, the more likely you are to develop a migraine. You may get a pounding migraine if you eat chocolate when you feel stressed, or when you drink coffee after a night of insomnia. If you get a migraine when you eat Parmesan or other aged cheeses, try eliminating these foods from your diet or eating them only in moderation. Ditto for big-screen movies, if flickering lights in a darkened theater set off your headaches. The best prescription for long-term relief does not come in a bottle; identifying and avoiding as many triggers as possible is key to effective self-management.

The right behavioral changes can help you manage your migraines. The headaches may not disappear—you remain susceptible to the triggers that cause them—but they will be less frequent and less intense. Adjusting your schedule so that you get up, eat, exercise, and go to bed at about the same time each day will reboot your *circadian rhythm* (your internal body clock that regulates the 24-hour cycle of biological processes), removing many of the disruptions that can activate migraines. Relieving stress and avoiding other contributing behaviors can bring about enormous improvement. Stress is one of the major contributors to migraine, but it is also something that can be managed. Anger, anxiety, and similar emotions release chemicals in the brain that may lead to migraines.

Over-the-counter analgesics work well for acute pain, but they are

RETHINKING MIGRAINE TRIGGERS

Migraine sufferers are often advised to avoid chocolate, red wine, aged cheeses, caffeine, and other foods that are suspected causes. But we are now beginning to realize that these foods themselves may not be triggers for headaches. Instead, it may be that physiological changes in the body during the premonitory phase of a migraine cause cravings for these foods and sensitivity to them.

usually weak weapons against migraines. Taken immediately at onset, migraine-specific medications are more efficient. Ergotamines (Cafergot, Migranal) have been used for years to treat migraine, but the tradeoff for pain relief comes at a cost: they can cause nausea, vomiting, muscle cramping, and other unpleasant side effects. Triptans, the first medications developed specifically for migraines, are the treatment standard. Sumatriptan (Imitrex), zolmitriptan (Zomig), almotriptan (Axert), and other triptans relieve pain for some (but not all) migraine sufferers without the side effects of ergotamines; some people who use them experience tingling, drowsiness, or flushing. Some trial-and-error effort may be necessary to find which triptan is most effective.

Other approaches work well for some people. If you have migraines more than four times per month, preventive medications, including antidepressants and anticonvulsants, may help to reduce the frequency and strength of your headaches. Botulinum toxin (Botox) is another alternative if you have migraines for 15 or more days per month. Injections at 12-week or longer intervals, at several locations on the head and neck, greatly decrease the intensity and frequency of headaches.[6] In the most severe cases, an implantable nerve stimulator (discussed in chapter 5) may be the only way to achieve adequate relief from disabling daily headaches, including migraines.

Tension-Type Headaches

Most adults have occasional *tension-type headaches* (formerly referred to as "tension headaches"). Once thought to be the most common type of headache, many tension-type headaches, we now believe, are misdiagnosed migraines. It is easy to confuse the two, since some symptoms are similar and many people suffer from both kinds. The dominant symptom of tension-type headaches is mild to moderate aching that lasts for 30 minutes or several days on both sides of the head, although it may occur only on one side. Some people describe the pain as a tight band of pressure, as though their heads were gripped in a vice. Unlike throbbing migraines, tension-type headaches produce a steady pain that is sometimes accompanied by nausea. They are considered to be chronic when they appear on 15 or more days per month for several months.

We do not know whether tense muscles help trigger these changes or occur because of them. Muscle contractions were long thought to be the cause, but studies show no evidence that the muscles covering the skull contract during painful tension-type headaches. Researchers now hypothesize that tension-type headaches and migraines may be caused by unknown chemical functions in the brain; people who have depression or sleep disorders tend to develop tension-type headaches from fluctuating levels of serotonin and other neurotransmitters that activate pain pathways in the brain. Stress, fatigue, eyestrain, poor vision, and other behavioral actions can also act as triggers, another similarity with migraines.

Tension-type headaches do not normally interfere with routine activities and are resolved with over-the-counter analgesics. They can be dramatically improved by a combination of the following:

- stress management, including biofeedback therapy
- physical therapy
- limiting headache medications
- limiting caffeine intake

- regulating sleep and exercise
- correcting vision problems
- correcting teeth grinding

Spinal Headaches

Although rare, *spinal headaches* are caused when needles used in epidural or lumbar procedures puncture the *dura,* the thin membrane surrounding and containing the spinal fluid. If the fluid that normally surrounds the spinal cord and cushions the brain leaks, subtle pressure changes may trigger extremely painful headaches. Posture is a telltale symptom: lying prone provides instant relief, while standing or sitting is more painful. Spinal headache pain at the back or front of the head may range from mild to excruciating and may be accompanied by nausea, reduced hearing, ringing in the ears, double vision, neck pain, or sensitivity to light. Bed rest for a few days is necessary. Hydration is important to increase production of spinal fluid, and intravenous fluids may be recommended. Caffeine may also provide temporary relief. Spinal headaches typically disappear when the dural leak heals spontaneously. If they persist after 48 hours, an anesthesiologist may administer a *blood patch*. This involves injecting a small amount of blood taken from the arm into the epidural space so that the resulting clot of blood seals the leak. This treatment works most of the time within a few hours; a second blood patch is sometimes required.

Low-Back Pain and Neck Pain

Up to 80 percent of the U.S. population have back pain sooner or later. It is one of the leading causes of disability in people under age 45, second only to the common cold. Chronic back pain develops from aging, arthritis, and other degenerative diseases of the discs and joints and can be symptomatic of other conditions. Most lower-back pain results from lifting or moving in a way that strains the back. The resulting acute pain can be uncomfortable, but it is normally controlled with over-the-counter medications, massage, or applications of heat or cold until the injury heals on its own. Every effort should be made to rapidly bring intense lower-back pain under control before it becomes chronic. Physical therapy is often a key element of treatment.

Disc Damage

Gel-filled discs act as shock absorbers between the bony vertebrae that form the spine. Healthy discs create flexibility in the spine, allowing it to twist and bend forward and backward. Discs degenerate as we age, becoming thinner and drying out until they shrink and no longer provide adequate cushioning between the bones. A *bulging disc,* which usually develops gradually, protrudes beyond its normal position. *Herniated discs* (also referred to as *ruptured* or *slipped discs*) occur when a portion of the interior gel leaks into the spinal canal through a crack in the outer layer of the disc (figure 2.1). Herniated discs typically develop suddenly

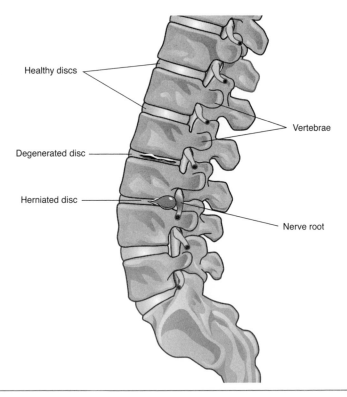

FIGURE 2.1. Pain can develop in the back, arms, and legs when a damaged or deteriorated disc presses on a nearby nerve root.

as a result of an injury to the spine, but they are not always painful. In fact, many people are unaware of the problem until it shows up on magnetic resonance imaging (MRI). A protruding disc can press on a nerve root, triggering radiating pain and numbness in the back and down the leg. A herniated disc in the neck acts in the same way, sending pain signals down the arm. If medication or rest does not resolve the problem, it may be appropriate to consider injections of steroids into the surrounding epidural space. Minimally invasive procedures can also remove some or all of the disc material to relieve pressure on the nerve root.

Degenerated discs sometimes collapse so extensively they cause *spinal stenosis* (table 2.2), a narrowing of the spinal canal, which contains sensitive nerves. The condition may not cause any symptoms if the narrowed spinal canal does not compress nerves that provide sensation to the back and legs. Nerves that become compressed, however, can produce excruciating pain. *Lumbar stenosis* (in the lower back) and *cervical stenosis* (in the neck) often develop gradually as we get older, generally after age 50. Stenosis occurs sooner in people with inherited spinal ab-

TABLE 2.2 Symptoms of stenosis

Lumbar stenosis	Cervical stenosis
Low-back pain	Pain in the neck or shoulders
Pain radiating into the buttocks and legs	Pain radiating into the arms and hands
Numbness, tingling, or weakness in one or both legs	Numbness, tingling, or weakness in one or both hands
Pain relieved by sitting or bending forward	Initial pain may be limited to certain positions of the neck and arms
Pain worse when walking or standing for long periods	If severe, may cause *spasticity* (difficulty walking or controlling the legs)

normalities and those who have an injury, tumor, scoliosis, osteoarthritis, or other degenerative spinal condition. *Cauda equina syndrome* is caused by extreme compression of the nerves in the lower spine. This is a serious condition that requires surgery to prevent paralysis and permanent loss of bowel and bladder control.

Lumbar Facet Joint Pain

Deteriorated lumbar facet joints—the interlocking paired joints between and behind vertebrae that stabilize the spine and facilitate movement—cause a high percentage of chronic low-back pain. The lumbar portion of the spine (the lower part), the most flexible part, supports most of the body's weight, making it particularly prone to damage and deterioration. When facet joints are injured or become worn down, the sensory nerves in the joint lining create a barrage of pain signals. This type of pain is often misdiagnosed as a herniated disc, since symptoms of both conditions are similar. Lumbar facet joint pain, however, is usually intermittent and more pronounced when a person leans backward.

Chronic facet joint pain sometimes responds to conservative self-management: applying heat and cold, using anti-inflammatories, staying active, and practicing good posture. The next step is physical therapy and more potent analgesics. For persistent cases, nerves around the facet joints can be deadened with a needle-based procedure known as a *facet rhizotomy*. After a local anesthetic is administered, an x-ray-guided needle is positioned adjacent to the affected facet joint. An electrode at the tip of the needle is then heated, killing the nerves so that pain signals cannot progress to the brain. If severe pain persists, it may be necessary to fuse two adjacent vertebrae. Nerves do regrow, so facet rhizotomies commonly need to be repeated after 9 to 12 months.

Nerve Damage

Sciatica is pain that extends from the buttock down one leg when spinal nerve roots leading to the sciatic nerve (the largest nerve in the body) become pinched. Any sudden movement, even a cough or a sneeze, can send mild to intense burning, aching, or throbbing pains shooting down the leg, making it painful to sit, stand, or walk. Many people with sciatica find that using an ergonomically designed chair helps when sitting. If the nerve between the disc and the bone is pinched, people experience numbness and some weakness in the leg. Most often, a herniated disc or spinal stenosis is the problem.

If NSAIDs and special exercises fail to control sciatic pain, muscle relaxants, deep tissue massage, or ultrasound treatment may be recommended. (See a video of three sciatica exercises at the SpineUniverse website, www.spineuniverse.com/conditions/sciatica/exercises-sciatica -herniated-disc.) Many people who have sciatica find yoga, tai chi, aqua therapy, and acupuncture helpful. Similarly, chiropractic therapy may help to relieve acute pain, but it is inadvisable for acute disc herniation or instability of the spine. Epidural steroid injections may provide relief by surrounding the inflamed nerve roots with anti-inflammatory medication. Several other newer, minimally invasive, disc procedures are promising, but their efficacy is not yet established.

Another nerve problem is painful *arachnoiditis,* which develops when the protective arachnoid membrane encircling nerves in the spinal cord becomes inflamed, creating scar tissue that binds nerves together. Twitching, cramping, tingling, numbness, or burning, stinging pain may develop when arachnoiditis impedes neural functionality. Treatment primarily consists of anti-inflammatory medications, to reduce swelling

Shakespeare was familiar with the disabling pain of sciatica. In his play *Timon of Athens* (act 4, scene 1), the main character rages against the city, cursing its inhabitants with misfortune and destruction. He says, "Thou cold sciatica, cripple our senators, that their limbs may halt as lamely as their manners."

and decrease pain, and neuropathic pain medications (see chapter 3).

Physical therapy, nerve blocks, and other treatments successfully manage mild to moderate back and neck pain. Steroid injections can subdue inflammation, but the pain tends to recur if the underlying problem is significant. For severe cases, surgery performed sooner rather than later is recommended if no progress is made after four to six months of treatment and if the back problem can be surgically repaired. A five-year multi-institution study found that surgery to remove part of the offending disc or vertebra provided faster relief, better physical function, and greater satisfaction for patients with herniated discs and spinal stenosis; it was the preferred treatment even among patients who had *spondylolisthesis*, a painful condition caused when a neck or lumbar vertebra slips forward out of alignment.[7] At this point, if the condition is severe, the only remaining treatment is usually surgical fusion that mechanically locks two or more vertebrae together.

Neck Pain

Neck pain can radiate into the shoulders and upper back and may cause headaches and tingling or numbness in the extremities. Rheumatoid arthritis, spinal stenosis, injury, poor posture, and degenerative disc disease may also compromise the structural integrity of discs, causing them to thin or flatten. Progressive cartilage deterioration from osteoarthritis is the most common cause of cervical facet joint pain. Loss of disc height may reposition the affected facet joints too close to each other, thereby disrupting normal functionality of the joint. Treatment includes physical therapy and steroid injections into the epidural space or directly into damaged facet joints. Pulsed radiofrequency can also be used for cervical facet rhizotomies. This newer technique temporarily "stuns" facet nerves to stop them from sending pain signals. (You will read more about this procedure in chapter 5.)

Other Chronic Neuropathic Pain Conditions

Chronic nerve pain can develop from bursitis, carpal tunnel syndrome, stroke, multiple sclerosis, and many other disorders. High levels of blood sugar associated with diabetes also damage blood vessels and nerves. Up to 70 percent of people who have diabetes have neuropathy pain in their hands, feet, arms, or legs. People who drink alcohol excessively are at greater risk for developing similar pain.

Complex Regional Pain Syndrome

Enduring pain can affect areas of the body beyond what is expected from a single injury. Unfamiliar to most people, *complex regional pain syndrome* (CRPS) produces such pain. Formerly referred to as reflex sympathetic dystrophy, CRPS is usually but not always triggered by an injury to a limb, but the pain is out of proportion to the initial injury. It is a classic example of neuropathic pain, with the nervous system signaling pain abnormally. It often affects a limb that has been in a cast or a sling or has been otherwise underused. For reasons we do not understand, the pain remains when the injury heals, perhaps because of an autoimmune response. CRPS runs in families and is more common among middle-aged people, but it also occurs in young people.

Diagnosing CRPS can be an exasperating process for the patient and the medical team. We understand more about it than ever before, but existing guidelines are broad and we still lack definitive diagnostic tools. Key criteria are clinical symptoms of nerve dysfunction and pain beyond what is expected for the injury. Other signs might include abrupt texture and temperature changes in the skin, which may become dry, flaky, sweaty, and shiny; or it may take on redness, a pallor, or blue mottling. Swelling or stiffness in the area and brittle or slow-growing nails may also develop. Muscles may become weak and stiff, and the affected hand or foot may jerk and twitch. Allodynia (painful sensitivity) is another signal that the nervous system is in high-alarm mode.

CRPS treatment is difficult, but thankfully, we can curtail the suffering of many persons who have CRPS. The most effective strategy is to attack the syndrome on multiple fronts, using anti-inflammatories and low-dose opioids to take the edge off the pain. Anticonvulsants, antidepressants, and nerve blocks can dramatically reduce abnormal sensitivity. These medications repress the pain enough that the person can pursue physical therapy, which desensitizes the painful area to touch, pressure, and movement. People who do not respond well to this approach may benefit from electrical stimulation of the affected nerves from a surgically implanted device. Stress management is also important, to counteract triggers that activate the sympathetic nervous system and increase muscle tension, which in turn amplifies pain. *Bisphosphonates,* a class of drugs used to treat osteoporosis and cancer-related bone pain, and infusions of ketamine, a potent anesthetic that alters central sensitization, may be potential treatments for CRPS. Both drug treatments significantly reduced pain levels in preliminary trials. Much more research is necessary to determine the safety, effectiveness, and applicable doses of these medications.[8]

Shingles

If you have ever had chicken pox, the varicella-zoster virus that causes it remains dormant in your nerves. The virus sometimes reactivates for unknown reasons, causing *herpes zoster infection* (shingles). Anyone who has had chicken pox may later develop shingles, especially when nerve cells are stimulated by a weakened immune system. Shingles can be maddening and incredibly painful. Burning or tingling pain, which can be severe, usually precedes blisters and a rash. Some people also experience fever or chills, joint pain, swollen lymph nodes, or abdominal pain. The blisters and rash are almost always limited to one side of the body, and they normally disappear within 90 days, even without treatment.

Treatment with acyclovir or other antiviral medication within 72 hours of the first symptom is crucial to reduce the risk of *postherpetic neuralgia* (PHN), which develops from nerve damage and remains after the symptoms of shingles disappear. PHN is not always terribly painful, but it can produce sharp stabbing or burning pain that may calm after several months or may evolve into chronic pain. Treatment may include over-the-counter antihistamines for itching and capsaicin cream, nerve blocks, or narcotics to manage pain. Anticonvulsants and antidepressant medications also help to minimize pain and improve the person's sleep. The doctor may prescribe a numbing lidocaine patch or a high-dose capsaicin patch (Qutenza), which is administered in the office after the skin is anesthetized. The Centers for Disease Control recommends a shingles vaccine (Zostavax) for people age 60 and older, including those who have previously had shingles. The vaccine reduces the risk of developing shingles by half and decreases the severity of the illness in those who will still develop shingles; the vaccine is not recommended for individuals with weakened immune systems, however.

Myofascial Pain

Muscle injury and abnormal strain from poor posture, occupational activities, and sports can cause *myofascial trigger points.* These hypersensitive areas in the muscles can sometimes cause tender knots that can be felt under the skin and may develop into sources of chronic pain. Emotional stress may also aggravate trigger points.

Myofascial pain is sometimes mistaken for fibromyalgia, but the two conditions produce different pain patterns (a person may have either or both conditions). Fibromyalgia creates widespread pain, while myofascial pain is localized in the area of the trigger point; myofascial trigger points also sometimes produce *referred pain,* pain that is felt in another area of the body. Treatment options may include anti-inflammatory med-ications, chiropractic care, and physical therapy to relieve tension. Myo-fascial release, a type of gentle deep tissue massage, may also be effective. When other therapies are inadequate, *trigger-point injections* of a local anesthetic given directly into the troubled area may relieve the pain. If you have more than one trigger point, several injections can be given during a single visit to your doctor. Unresponsive trigger points may gradually relax after botulinum toxin injections. If you are allergic to the medications, a *dry-needle* procedure can be performed: a needle without medication is used to apply direct pressure to the trigger point.

Chronic Pelvic Pain

Chronic pelvic pain is a common problem among women that is often overlooked and underdiagnosed. It may be caused by current or past infections or by *endometriosis,* which is growth of the endometrial lining (the same tissue that is shed during menstruation) beyond its normal location in the uterus and into the ovaries, the bowels, or other pelvic tissues. Chronic endometriosis and other causes of chronic inflamma-tion may cause pain during menstruation and intercourse and may result in persistent back pain. These conditions can also affect fertility. Treat-ment may include NSAIDs and hormone therapy. When the pain is ex-treme, surgery may be tried, although it is a last resort.

Men also suffer from chronic pelvic pain. In fact, it is the most com-mon reason males under age 50 consult with a urologist. *Chronic pelvic pain syndrome* (CPPS) causes unexplained discomfort at the base of the penis, in the testicles, or in the rectum. The pain may be greater during urination, bowel movements, sex, or when sitting for long periods. Some men with CPPS also develop erectile dysfunction. CPPS is sometimes referred to as chronic prostatitis, but this is somewhat of a misnomer, since the prostate is not always inflamed or painful. Stress-induced pelvic spasms that continually tense the muscles are thought to cause CPPS—90 percent of men diagnosed with the condition have this type of spasming. Conventional therapies, including analgesics and anti-inflammatories, counteract symptomatic pain. Symptoms also respond to pelvic-floor relaxation exercises and pressure massage of hypersensitive muscle knots by a trained therapist.[9]

Phantom Pain

Hundreds of thousands of people in the United States who have had limbs amputated suffer with persistent *phantom pain.* Very real and sometimes unbearable, phantom pain is felt in a part of the body that no longer exists. (This is not the same as *stump pain,* which is pain at the point of amputation.) Phantom pain can also develop in areas that lose sensation after stroke or paralysis, yet it almost universally occurs in limb amputees, perhaps because the brain retains the memory of pain and keeps sending pain signals after the limb is removed. One theory is that areas of the brain process missing limbs differently: the portion of the brain responsible for thinking recognizes that the body part is gone, yet the feeling part of the brain "remembers" the relative position of the missing part. Pain that is poorly controlled during an amputation may also be a cause. Evidence suggests that the chance of developing phantom pain is decreased when regional anesthesia is used to provide thorough pain relief prior to surgery and for the first few postoperative days.[10]

Some persons itch in the missing part or feel cramping; others experience harsh pain. The symptoms may resolve in a few months, but often they turn into a classic case of chronic nerve pain. Although neuropathic pain medications can be useful, no single approach succeeds with all patients. In some people, nerve blocks and stump revision work well. Multidisciplinary treatment that is customized for each individual is the most effective.

Stimulation of the intact opposite limb has been shown to help rid patients of phantom pain and decrease the need for medication. *Mirror therapy,* a technique that is widely used by the military for people who have lost limbs during combat, is surprisingly effective. Patients hold their stump up to the backside of a mirror while they move their healthy limb in front of it. Observing the reflection of the healthy limb moving produces an optical illusion, as if the missing limb were moving. Repeating this process daily for several weeks tricks the brain into thinking that the missing limb is functional, which lessens pain and resolves the issue for some people. Some studies have shown that the same treatment decreases pain and enhances motor function in people who have early-stage CRPS or stroke-related pain.[11]

Irritable Bowel Syndrome

Another source of chronic pain with unidentified causes is *irritable bowel syndrome* (IBS), a common chronic intestinal disorder that affects twice as many women as men. Anxiety appears to be an exacerbating factor. IBS may be triggered by atypical signals sent between the brain and especially sensitive intestinal nerves. Symptoms include mild to chronic bloating, abdominal gas and cramping, and pain several days each month. People with IBS may have recurrent constipation, diarrhea, or alternating bouts of both. Loss of appetite is also common. Treatment consists mainly of behavioral and dietary changes combined with relaxation techniques to improve the symptoms, which can be disabling if they are not well managed. For many people, managing the symptoms is a lifelong effort.

Inflammatory Bowel Disease

Chronic ulceritis and Crohn's disease are types of *inflammatory bowel disease* (IBD). Chronic colitis affects the large intestine (colon), while Crohn's disease can develop in any part of the gastrointestinal tract. Both disorders create varying levels of abdominal stress and are capable of producing inflammation, bloating, cramping, and extreme pain that tends to wax and wane in intensity. The cause of IBD remains undiscovered, but it appears to be linked to changes in the communication between the nervous system, the brain, and the gastrointestinal tract.

Chronic Fatigue Syndrome

It is not surprising that *chronic fatigue syndrome* (CFS) causes long-lasting pain, since it simultaneously stresses all of the body's systems and functions. CFS is thought to be closely related to fibromyalgia. People with CFS feel utterly exhausted yet do not improve even when they get plenty of rest. They may suffer from gastrointestinal pain, have sore muscles and joints, and feel too cold, too hot, or dizzy. They may also be overly sensitive to sounds, lights, and smells and may experience diminished memory and cognitive abilities.

We have many theories about the potential causes of CFS, yet we lack definitive information about what happens in the body to create such a baffling disorder. The onset is often preceded by acute infection, leading some researchers to believe that latent pathogens in the body may affect the central nervous system. It is possible that these pathogens, which survive by infecting a host cell, become chronic at some point, creating CFS. Preliminary evidence suggests that *enteroviruses,* common viruses that enter the body through the gastrointestinal tract, may somehow be implicated—people who have CFS commonly have recurring gastrointestinal disorders, and many have irritable bowel syndrome. Analysis of stomach biopsies from people with CFS showed that 82 percent had at least one protein associated with an enterovirus.[12]

Numerous researchers have long suspected a relationship between CFS and the herpes family of viruses: Epstein-Barr (one of the most common viruses in humans), human herpesvirus 6 (HHV6), and cytomegalovirus. Martin Lerner, president of the Treatment Center for CFS, observed that many of his CFS patients also had one of these viruses. He conducted a compelling blind, randomized study to determine whether CFS patients would benefit from long-term antiviral treatment. Lerner and his colleagues divided 142 CFS patients with herpes-related infections into two groups: those with herpesvirus alone, and those who were coinfected with herpesvirus and another infection. All participants were treated with antiviral medications: those with Epstein-Barr received valacyclovir (Valtrex); others who had HHV6 or cytomegalovirus were given valganciclovir (Valcyte). Symptoms in about 75 percent of the patients in the herpesvirus-only group receded noticeably, so that individuals were able to resume a normal or near-normal lifestyle. The other group did not fare as well. They began the trial with more symptoms and were less affected by the treatment.[13]

To summarize, CFS is a perplexing and painful condition that includes all of the following:

- severe fatigue that lasts for six months or more and is not resolved with rest
- no indication of underlying disease
- at least four other specific simultaneous symptoms that occur during or after the development of severe fatigue, including muscle or joint pain, tender lymph nodes, sore throat, non-refreshing sleep, and headaches that were not experienced regularly before the fatigue occurred

Postoperative Pain

Despite the best efforts to aggressively treat pain during and after an operation, many patients develop chronic pain as a result of surgery. Postoperative pain is more likely in older patients and those who also have chronically painful conditions. It may develop when nerves are stretched, nicked, or otherwise damaged during a surgical procedure. Some pain may also result from scar tissue that naturally forms after surgery and may entrap or compress nerves. Radiation, chemotherapy, and other medical treatments may also exacerbate postoperative pain.

Adequate anesthesia during surgery and pain management during recovery is especially important—a greater level of pain experienced before and during surgery will likely result in more postsurgical pain.

Cancer surgery is capable of producing resistant pain. Many women who lose their breasts to cancer develop *postmastectomy pain syndrome,* a poorly studied and often misdiagnosed condition that occurs as sensory nerves in the chest are severed when breast tissue is removed. *Lymphedema* is another chronic condition that becomes painful when fluid builds up in a limb after lymph nodes are removed or following radiation therapy.

SUMMARY POINTS

- Numerous health conditions cause chronic pain.
- The causes of many chronically painful conditions are unknown.
- Neuropathic pain is the most challenging to diagnose and treat.
- A multidisciplinary approach is the one that most effectively treats chronic pain, regardless of the cause.

Pain Medications and How They Work

In a perfect world, relieving pain would involve a single dose of medication that would whisk away all traces of pain without unwanted side effects. But we do not live in a perfect world, and no panacea exists to counteract all the various causes and types of chronic pain. We do, however, have an impressive arsenal of analgesic tools to relieve or stop pain.

Although we don't have the perfect antidote for all types of pain, we have certainly come a long way since the time when physicians cut a hole in patients to "let the pain out." When you sprain an ankle, develop a headache, or spend too much time working in the yard, you need only to reach for the medicine cabinet to find a quick-acting tablet that alleviates your pain. Treating chronic pain is far more intricate, because no single analgesic or dose works for all people or against all types of pain. Side effects and drug interactions ranging from mildly uncomfortable to fatal must be carefully managed. Duration is another significant distinction between analgesics for acute and chronic pain. Many chronic pain sufferers need long-term medication, potentially for the remainder of their lives. While optimum pain management includes psychotherapy, physical therapy, and other approaches, analgesics are a mainstay for chronic pain treatment.

Pain medications work by reducing the frequency or intensity of pain signals sent to the brain or by modifying the way the brain perceives pain messages. Analgesics are most effective when they address the unique nuances of an individual's pain. It is also important to treat anxiety, depression, disrupted sleep, and other symptoms that often go hand in hand with chronic pain, because improving one symptom often greatly improves another.

Acetaminophen

Sold both over the counter and by prescription, acetaminophen relieves the discomfort of arthritis, fibromyalgia, and many other types of acute and chronic pain. It is frequently combined with aspirin and caffeine in migraine medications. Scientists are not quite sure how acetaminophen works. They suspect it modulates pain messages in the spinal cord and the brain to create greater pain tolerance. Used as directed, acetaminophen is usually well tolerated and side effects are rare. Taking too much can be harmful to the liver and even fatal—unintentional acetaminophen overdose is a serious problem in the United States. Large doses represent the greatest risk, but small amounts over a long period can also do harm. Drinking three or more servings of alcohol in 24 hours while taking acetaminophen also heightens the risk.

Acetaminophen is the active ingredient in hundreds of common medications used for colds, fever, allergies, and headaches, and overdose can occur more readily than you might think unless you carefully read labels. Look for "acetaminophen" or "APAP" on the list of ingredients, and make sure that the combined amount in all medications you take does

TABLE 3.1 Sample of products containing acetaminophen

Over-the-counter products	Prescription products
Anacin*	Endocet
Dayquil*	Esgic
Dristan*	Fioricet
Excedrin	Hydrocet
Midol*	Lortab
Nyquil*	Percocet
Pamprin*	Sedapap
Theraflu	Tylenol with codeine
Triaminic*	Ultracet
Tylenol	Vicodin
	Zydone

Note: Many other products are sold as generic and store brands.

*Some, but not all, formulations in product line contain acetaminophen.

not exceed the recommended dose according to package information or what your physician prescribes. Avoid taking more than one acetaminophen product at a time (table 3.1).

Nonsteroidal Anti-inflammatories

Nonsteroidal anti-inflammatory drugs (NSAIDs) are analgesic workhorses that reduce mild to moderate pain, inflammation, and fever. Patients who still have significant pain with over-the-counter NSAIDs may benefit from prescription combinations of NSAIDs and other medications. All NSAIDs have an analgesic threshold. A minimum amount is required for a medication to work, but at some point increasing the dose does not continue to increase effectiveness. Taking larger doses does not necessarily give more pain relief and is more likely to cause gastrointestinal damage. For most people, over-the-counter NSAIDs are safe for the occasional headache or back pain, but they can be problematic when used extensively or in high doses. Taking them for more than a few months is a balancing act between the benefit of reduced pain and the increased risk of serious side effects.

NSAIDs can cause severe allergic reactions (particularly in people with asthma) and elevate blood pressure (especially in people who already have high blood pressure). More than occasional use (even short-term use in some people) can cause ulcers and gastrointestinal bleeding. They also raise the risk for kidney damage, particularly in individuals who are dehydrated or have kidney disease. Controlled doses are safe for people who are not already at risk for these conditions. Elderly patients are particularly sensitive to NSAIDs and are more likely to take other medications that interact poorly. Anyone who is over age 65 or has kidney disease and takes an NSAID for more than six months should be monitored carefully for early signs of kidney damage. People with frequent acid reflux or heartburn should take an anti-acid medication (such as Prilosec or Prevacid) before using an NSAID and should consult with their doctor if they are taking more than four or five NSAID doses per month.

NSAIDs have different degrees of cardiovascular safety, which must be considered when choosing appropriate treatment. People with high risk or a history of heart attack or stroke should never use NSAIDs for any length of time. A landmark Danish study of 1 million healthy individuals who had at least one prescribed NSAID during a nine-year period found that common NSAIDs significantly increased the risk of stroke: by about 30 percent with ibuprofen and naproxen, and 86 percent with diclofenac. Doses of more than 1,200 milligrams per day raised the risk for heart attack; low doses appeared to decrease the risk. Naproxen (Aleve, Naprosyn) did not appear to affect the risk for either heart disease or stroke. Study authors found that rofecoxib (a drug no longer available in the United States) and diclofenac were associated with increased cardiovascular mortality and illness and should be used with caution in most individuals. Later Danish research reviewed subsequent use of NSAIDs by 99,187 people over the age of 30 who had first-time heart attacks. Researchers concluded that NSAIDs raised the risk for another coronary event, no matter how much time had elapsed since the first heart attack.[1] Analysis of more than 8,000 Taiwanese people also found that ibuprofen and other NSAIDs significantly raised the incidence of heart attack.[2]

Aspirin

Aspirin is the one drug most households are likely to have on hand. No other medication compares as an all-in-one reliever for mild to moderate aches, pain, fever, and inflammation. Over-the-counter and prescription-strength aspirin, which is often combined with other prescription medications (table 3.2), are often used in the short term for osteoarthritis, rheumatoid arthritis, migraines, and the painful side effects of other chronic conditions. For millions of people who have had a heart attack or have elevated risk for heart disease, aspirin is also a lifesaver: a single daily aspirin reduces the risk of cardiovascular events by thinning the blood and decreasing platelet clotting. It also reduces the risk of recurring stroke caused by a blood clot. Other NSAIDs also thin the blood, but unlike aspirin, once the drug is flushed from the system, blood consistency returns to normal; aspirin's effect may last for more than a week.

Aspirin works against pain by inhibiting production of prostaglandins, chemicals in the body that encourage inflammation and send pain messages to the brain when tissue is injured. Inexpensive and versatile,

TABLE 3.2 Sample of products containing aspirin

Over-the-counter products	Prescription products
Acuprin	Empirin with Codeine
Alka-Seltzer	Fiorinal
Anacin*	Halfprin
Ascriptin	Norgesic
Aspergum	Percodan
Aspirtab	
Bufferin	
Ecotrin	
Excedrin	
Pamprin*	

Note: Many other products are sold as generic and store brands.
*Some, but not all, formulations in product line contain aspirin.

aspirin is not perfect. Taking too much can diminish other "good" prostaglandins in the stomach, causing ulcers and stomach irritation.

Ibuprofen

Recommended for mild to moderate pain, ibuprofen (table 3.3), particularly in prescription strength, is often used for migraines, osteoarthritis,
and rheumatoid arthritis. Like other NSAIDs, it acts quickly. Common
side effects include nausea, dizziness, rash, and heartburn. Long-term
use and high doses can create stomach and kidney problems; because it
does not remain in the body for long, the risk for these complications is
less than with other NSAIDs. A new formulation of ibuprofen combined
with famotidine, a medicine used to treat ulcers and acid reflux, is showing promise for people who take NSAIDs for chronic pain and inflammation. Double-blind randomized studies at the University of Southern
California's Keck School of Medicine found that patients who took this
formulation (Duexis) three times daily had significantly fewer gastrointestinal ulcers than those who took ibuprofen alone.[3]

TABLE 3.3 **TABLE 3.3** **Sample of products containing ibuprofen**

Advil	Genpril	Motrin
Combunox	Ibudone	Nuprin
Duexis	Medipren	Reprexain
Dristan Sinus	Midol*	Vicoprofen

Note: Many other products are sold as generic and store brands.
*Some, but not all, formulations in product line contain ibuprofen.

COX-2 Inhibitors

NSAIDs reduce pain and inflammation by blocking cyclooxygenase-2 (COX-2) enzymes that create pain-inducing prostaglandins, but they also block protective COX-1 enzymes in the stomach. COX-2 inhibitors are selective second-generation NSAIDs developed to block only COX-2 enzymes. They reduce pain as effectively as other NSAIDs with less potential for gastric bleeding and ulcers, but they carry greater risk for heart attack and stroke (table 3.4). Celecoxib (Celebrex) is the only COX-2 still available in the United States. Rofecoxib (Vioxx) and valdecoxib (Bextra) were recalled because of concerns about their side effects. Since 2008, the Standard Care versus Celecoxib Outcome Trial, a collaborative effort of health clinicians in Denmark, the Netherlands, and the United King-

TABLE 3.4 **Risk indicators of COX-2 inhibitors and other nonsteroidal anti-inflammatory drugs (NSAIDs)**

Personal characteristic	Effect of NSAIDs	Effect of COX-2 inhibitors
Older	Raise risk of gastrointestinal problems	Less risk
Heavy drinker	Raise risk of gastrointestinal problems	Less risk
Taking steroids for asthma, arthritis, or other condition	Raise risk of gastrointestinal problems	Less risk
History of ulcers	Raise risk of gastrointestinal problems	Less risk
High risk or history of heart disease	Raise risk of heart disease	Greater risk
High risk or history of stroke	Raise risk of stroke	Greater risk

Note: Regular long-term use of most NSAIDs raises the risk for heart attack and stroke in healthy individuals.

dom, has been tracking the long-term effects of COX-2 inhibitors compared to other NSAIDs among arthritis patients. Results of this long-term investigation should help to clarify the effects of celecoxib on the cardiovascular system compared to other NSAIDs.

Opioids

Traditionally used for cancer-related pain or acute pain during post-operational recovery, opioids are increasingly recommended by pain specialists when other analgesics and therapies fail to provide adequate pain relief. Opioids are natural or synthetic drugs related to morphine, the gold standard for treating moderate to severe chronic pain. Opioids in various forms—pills, syrups, anal suppositories, injections, intravenous applications, and skin patches—make life easier for countless people who live with debilitating pain. Opioids are not appropriate or even effective for everyone, and not all individuals with chronic pain need them. For some, they provide a level of functioning that outweighs the negative side effects and risks. They are potentially dangerous at high doses, particularly for individuals who are extremely sensitive to their effects. Many persons who have chronic pain do very well with small doses; individuals with severe pain may need stronger opioids or a higher dose. As is the case with all medications, the smallest dose that provides adequate pain relief with manageable side effects is the right prescription for a person who needs opioids. While some side effects can be managed,

- *Narcotic* is a legal term for a controlled substance.
- Opium is a mind-altering powder derived from the seedpod of the *Papaver somniferum* poppy.
- Opiates are drugs made from opium.
- Opioids are natural or synthetic drugs that bind to opioid receptors and have qualities similar to those of morphine. The term *opioids* includes the opiates.

identifying just the right dose is key. Finding the right balance is part of the trial-and-error process.

Oxycodone, the opioid most commonly prescribed for chronic pain, is more potent than morphine. Taken in low doses, it is often effective against bone and nerve pain and has few unwanted side effects. Fentanyl skin patches and lozenges use very small amounts of fentanyl, since it is 100 times as strong as morphine. Transdermal patches containing buprenorphine (Butrans) can also be used to control moderate to severe pain and may have fewer side effects. Buprenorphine (Butrans, Subutex, Suboxone) appears to be well tolerated, with a low level of physical dependence and fewer withdrawal symptoms when it is stopped.[4] Methadone, an inexpensive and effective opioid that reduces withdrawal symptoms in addicts, is also used for chronic pain, especially when a slow-onset, long-acting opioid is needed. As a pain treatment, methadone reduces both tolerance and nerve super-sensitivity. It blocks N-methyl-D-aspartate (NMDA) receptors in the spinal cord, reducing the volume or intensity of pain signals that are transmitted by the spinal cord to the brain. Methadone must be used cautiously because its long half-life (the time it takes for the body to clear one-half of the drug out of the body) can lead to dangerously high accumulations in the blood.

Opioids are classified as agonists, antagonists, or a combination of both. Opioid agonists (morphine and methadone) activate mu opioid receptors (chemical receptors on nerves that regulate pain) in the central nervous system. Like endorphins, agonists act like brakes on pain pathways. Buprenorphine and some other opioids are partial agonists; they bind only to a portion of the mu receptors, but they may bind to other types of opioid receptors, providing limited pain relief. Opioid antagonists (naltrexone, naloxone) also bind to receptors, but they do not elicit a response. They simply take up space that otherwise would be used by pain-reducing opioids or endorphins. Tapentadol and tramadol have opioid effects and elevate the levels of serotonin and norepinephrine in the nervous system, subduing pain messages and lowering the brain's perception of pain. Antagonists are used primarily for addiction to alcohol or opioids or to reverse the effects of an opioid overdose, and they are sometimes prescribed off-label (legally prescribed in a way that is not included in the Food and Drug Administration's approval of the drug) to treat fibromyalgia, Crohn's disease, and other painful inflammatory conditions. Agonist-antagonist medicines (pentazocine, butorphanol) work both ways. The agonist component of the medication reduces pain, and the antagonist portion has been thought to limit respiratory depression, but this is unclear. Similar combination opioids are used for mild to moderate pain that does not require more potent medication.

If you have ever taken Vicodin (acetaminophen combined with hydrocodone) or Percocet (acetaminophen combined with oxycodone) after dental surgery, you have had an immediate-release opioid that acts quickly and then fades after three to four hours. Extended-release, or long-acting opioids (table 3.5), are prescribed for persistent, moderate to severe pain that requires long-term treatment. Compared to their immediate-release counterparts, many extended-release opioid medications keep a sustained

TABLE 3.5   Examples of long-acting opioids used for chronic pain

Drug	Brand names	Action
Buprenorphine	Buprenex, Butrans, Suboxone, Subutex	Long acting
Fentanyl	Duragesic	Extended release
Hydromorphone	Exalgo	Extended release
Methadone	Dolophine, Methadose	Long acting
Morphine	Avinza, Kadian, MS Contin, Oramorph	Extended release
Oxycodone	Oxycontin	Extended release
Oxymorphone	Opana ER	Extended release
Tapentadol	Nucynta ER	Extended release

level of analgesic in the blood, enabling a person to function better during the day and sleep better at night.

People who are new to opioids for pain management usually begin with codeine, hydrocodone, morphine, or other drugs with a short half-life. Depending on the characteristics and frequency of the pain, a low-dose mild opioid may provide relief. Individuals who respond well to short-half-life opioids and still have severe or persistent pain may need a stronger, extended-release opioid. Determining which opioid works best for an individual can require some effort. Some patients do better with a combination of both short-acting and long-acting opioids, or opioids combined with other pain medications.

◉ **BETTER PAIN CONTROL WITH THE RIGHT OPIOID**

PHIL'S BACK PAIN HAD GOTTEN WORSE AND WORSE until it was constant and severe and radiated into both of his legs. Unable to walk without pain, his functionality was greatly compromised, and as a result, his mental health and mood also suffered. An MRI showed that degenerative disc disease was the source of his pain. It was a situation that was unlikely to improve on its own, and the pain medications he had already tried were only somewhat helpful. On his doctor's recommendation, Phil proceeded with a laminectomy in hopes of regaining significant functionality. During the procedure, an orthopedic surgeon removed a portion of the vertebra above the offending disc to provide more space around the nerve root. Unfortunately, Phil's pain was no better after the procedure. In fact, it became worse, so his doctor recommended an anti-inflammatory, plus a combination of acetamin-ophen and immediate-release oxycodone. This prescription provided limited relief for three to four hours, but the pain always returned, so Phil needed more medication throughout the day.

When Phil came to us, we believed he would be better served by re-placing his oxycodone with an extended-release opioid. Taking the medi-cation just twice a day was easier, and it maintained a more consistent level of pain control. As a result, he no longer dreaded the wait for his medication to take effect or worried about its wearing off. The con-stant level of medication in his system managed Phil's pain with a lower dose, which he tolerated well. We also supplemented his opioid with a neuropathic pain medicine and recommended physical therapy and a gradually increasing exercise program. This overall strategy proved to be beneficial. Although his pain improved by only 30 percent, it was enough for him to recover a great deal of functionality, so that he was more active throughout the day and slept undisturbed during the night.

Side Effects of Opioids

All medications are double-edged swords with benefits and risks, and opioids are no exception. For many individuals, opioids are the difference between a life that is controlled by pain and a functional life with con-

GENETIC TESTING PREDICTS A MEDICATION'S EFFECTIVENESS

Although not yet in clinical use, predicting drug response based on a person's genetic markers is an early step in personalized medicine. With a simple blood sample or cheek swab, predictive testing can determine how individuals will respond to certain chemotherapies, clotting drugs, and other medications. Test results indicate which people will likely benefit from those medications and which ones probably will not. Those who test negatively thus can be spared the ordeal of treatments that would probably prove to be ineffective. Genetic testing can also help determine appropriate starting doses of morphine for patients with chronic pain. By identifying an individual's variation of the CYP2D6 gene, doctors can tell whether the patient can be expected to metabo-lize morphine slowly, quickly, or at all, and the medication can be prescribed accordingly.

WHEN OPIOIDS INCREASE PAIN SENSITIVITY

Anyone who takes opioids can gradually develop hyperalgesia, a heightened sensitivity to all painful stimuli. The condition is more prevalent in people who regularly take large doses or who were previously addicted. Decreasing or changing the type of opioid used or switching to a nonopioid medication usually resolves the issue.

trolled pain. Unlike NSAIDs and acetaminophen, opioids are not inherently toxic to organs; they do not cause gastrointestinal bleeding or raise blood pressure. Like all drugs, though, opioids can produce adverse side effects:

- Nausea or vomiting may occur, but it usually fades as an individual's system acclimates to the medication. If this side effect continues, a different opioid can be prescribed.
- Opioids bind to mu receptors in the intestinal tract, making constipation a common side effect that does not fade with ongoing use. Prophylactic management with laxatives, stool softeners, and increased fluid intake typically corrects the issue.
- Opioid-induced itching is mitigated with antihistamines.
- Reducing the dose usually controls drowsiness.
- Men who take opioids for an extended period may experience low testosterone levels, reduced libido, and erectile dysfunction.
- The stronger opioids can cause confusion, delirium, and dizziness. These symptoms can be brought to tolerable levels by reducing the dose or can be avoided altogether by changing the type of opioid.
- Depressed breathing is serious but rare at clinical doses. It is more likely with overdoses and with initial intravenous application, which should be closely monitored.

Controversy, Underuse, and Misunderstanding

Using opioids for chronic pain remains controversial, and sadly, many people who could benefit from them never have the opportunity. In the minds of many consumers, regulators, politicians, and even some physicians, "opioid" conjures images of bleary-eyed old men puffing on opium pipes in dark smoky rooms until they become oblivious to everything around them. The truth is that some opioids are quite powerful—that is what makes them so effective. Well-controlled studies over the past 20 years show that these medications are safe when used appropriately for pain; however, the efficacy of chronic opioid use is unclear. Opioids can be dangerous and even deadly when they are abused or misused: we have all heard news stories of celebrities who become addicted to pain pills, shuttle in and out of rehab, or die from overdoses or combining prescription drugs with alcohol.

Abuse and misuse of prescription pain relievers, including opioids, is an undeniable epidemic in this country. Enough prescription painkillers were prescribed in 2010 to medicate every American adult around the clock for an entire month. Prescription medications have replaced heroin and cocaine as the addict's drugs of choice. According to the Centers for Disease Control and Prevention, deaths from opioid overdoses more than tripled between 1999 and 2008, paralleling a 300 percent upswing of prescription opioids during the same period.[5] Drug abuse accounts for much of the problem; also contributing to abuse are patients who exceed their recommended doses, leave their medications where others can find them, or share them with others. Physicians are increasingly pressured to pay more attention to pain control, yet few are trained to understand or treat chronic pain or understand the nuances of various opioids. Federal regulations of prescription analgesics are more restrictive than ever, and as a result, many physicians fear overtreating patients. Others are apprehensive of government scrutiny or retribution for what may be considered prescribing powerful medications too freely. Some doctors ask patients to sign an opioid agreement to make sure they are aware of possible complications before taking these drugs.

What the media, the general public, and many doctors do not understand or appreciate is that repeatedly, studies show that opioids are safe and the risk of addiction is quite low when persons without prior addiction take them exactly as prescribed. According to the National Institutes of Health, about 5 percent of pain patients who take opioids over 12 months develop an addiction disorder.[6] An analysis of 26 studies involving almost 25,000 pain patients who took opioids found that many discontinued long-term use because of side effects and that only seven (about 0.03 percent) became addicted.[7] Elevated risk is certainly a greater issue for those who have a history of substance abuse. Being chemically dependent on a medication is dramatically different from being addicted to it. Addicts and people with chronic pain have dramatically different use profiles where opioids are concerned. Addicts do not adhere to prescribed doses. Desperate for a high, they may crush the tablets into powder, which they then snort or inject, sending dangerously high doses of the drug quickly through their bloodstream and into their brains. The result may be a fatal overdose. When opioids are given to people with addiction problems, their craving is amplified and their day-to-day functioning deteriorates. People taking opioids for pain, in contrast, report less pain and improved day-to-day functioning. Unlike addicts, whose lives become increasingly constricted by their obsession with drug use, people who are given opioids for pain tend to be able to expand the scope of their lives.

The Issue of Chemical Dependence

People who take opioids for pain rarely become psychologically addicted (table 3.6), but they often become physically dependent, meaning that their bodies become conditioned to expect the medication and would develop withdrawal symptoms if it was discontinued abruptly; that is why we carefully taper off opioids when they are to be stopped. Ideally, patients need less medication, including opioids, as they manage their pain with other modalities. Some patients take opioids for years without any adverse effects.

Tolerance is a separate issue that should not be confused with addiction. It refers to the need for larger doses of a drug to achieve the same effect. Patients develop tolerance with regular use and may need gradually increased doses to manage severe pain. Traditionally, scientists have agreed that tolerance occurs when the brain adapts to a drug's chemical compounds; we know that opioids alter the way receptors receive and metabolize these chemicals. Newer studies are fueling speculation that tolerance is actually a learned response resulting from specific internal

TABLE 3.6 Common myths about opioids

Opioid myths	Opioid facts
Opioids are dangerous	Opioids are safe when used as prescribed by a qualified physician
Opioids are addicting	People with no prior addiction who take opioids for pain rarely become addicted, although they may become physically tolerant and dependent
People who take opioids for pain get "high"	Low to modest doses of opioids used for pain do not generally create a sense of euphoria. Some people experience less pain because they have a general sense of well-being and relief from anxiety and depression
Taking opioids makes a person unresponsive and zombie-like	For most people, finding the right type of opioid at the most appropriate dose does not cause extreme sedation
Patients need increasing amounts of opioids to control pain	Doses usually stabilize in time; increases are needed only if pain levels increase
Opioids suppress all pain	Opioids do not eliminate new or different pain sensations

or environmental cues that are paired with administration of the drug. The implication could be significant for chronic pain sufferers who become tolerant of their medication: if drug tolerance can be learned, then it can also be unlearned, which could reduce or eliminate the need for greater, more powerful doses.

A project at the University of California illustrated that changes in environment—sights, sounds, smells, or colors that are present when medication is administered—can decrease tolerance, at least in lab rats. Rats were taken from their home cages each day and injected with the same amount of morphine by the same lab technician. The animals were then tested to see how well the drug blocked pain (technicians measured how much heat could be applied to each rat's tail before it moved away). After two weeks, rats that had become morphine tolerant were given their shot in a cage of a different color. Surprisingly, the medication worked as effectively as it did originally; the animals were no longer tolerant of the identical dose of the same medication.[8]

Your attitude affects how your pain meds work. We are often told not to underestimate the power of positive thinking; perhaps we should be equally cautious of negative expectations concerning pain medications. Volunteers who were told they would be subjected to a brief intense burning pain that would be relieved by an effective painkiller experienced the relief they expected. When researchers told them they would again be exposed to the burning without the medication, the volunteers experienced worse pain, even though they received the same amount of the same drug. The result is an example of the nocebo effect, a negative response brought about by a negative expectation.[9]

Adjunct Medications for Neuropathic Pain

Opioids and NSAIDs are traditional analgesic keystones, but they do not work as robustly for the complex nuances of neuropathic pain, one of the most frustrating types of pain to treat. Early recognition and aggressive management of neuropathic pain is critical to a successful outcome and calls for unique analgesic tools, including some that are used off-label.

Antidepressants

Many drugs originally developed for one treatment have been seren-dipitously discovered to be effective for something else. Such is the case with tricyclic antidepressants (TCAs), the oldest type of antidepressant medication and our first developed treatment for neuropathic pain. TCAs also relieve chronic nerve pain by decreasing feelings of depression and anxiety, but you need not have those feelings to realize the pain-reducing benefits.

We are not exactly sure how TCAs work as analgesics—they may in-crease pain-suppressing chemicals (serotonin and norepinephrine) in the spinal cord—but they often provide welcome relief from moderate pain of arthritis, migraine, fibromyalgia, and other chronic conditions. (Back pain may be different—a 2008 Cochrane review of 10 studies found no conclusive evidence that antidepressants are of significant benefit for back pain.)[10] Amitriptyline (Elavil), imipramine (Tofranil), and doxepin (Sinequan), in considerably lower doses than are used to treat depression, work well against steady burning or lancinating (sharp, stabbing) nerve pain and improve a person's quality of sleep. Taking the drugs in gradu-ally higher doses, most people experience mild, manageable side effects: drowsiness, constipation, and dry mouth. Some people gain weight or have difficulty urinating while taking TCAs.

Chronic neuropathic pain is also treated with two other types of anti-depressants. Serotonin and norepinephrine reuptake inhibitors (SNRIs), including venlafaxine (Effexor) and duloxetine (Cymbalta), are helpful for some people with musculoskeletal pain and neuropathic pain. SNRIs may be less effective than TCAs, but they cause fewer side effects. Duloxetine is Food and Drug Administration (FDA) approved to treat depression, anxiety, fibromyalgia, diabetic neuropathy, and chronic musculoskeletal pain. Two well-designed studies show that it also reduces osteoarthritis knee pain when taken alone or in combination with NSAIDs. In both projects, participants who took duloxetine for 13 weeks reported 33 per-cent greater pain relief than those who took a placebo during the same period; some of the duloxetine patients reported that their pain levels were decreased by 50 percent or more.[11] Another study, a 10-week clinical trial involving 524 patients who were already taking NSAIDs for moderate or severe pain from osteoarthritis of the knee, concluded that the addition of duloxetine reduced pain and improved function better than NSAIDs combined with a placebo.[12] Other investigations support the use of duloxetine for diabetic peripheral neuropathic pain, fibromyalgia, and chronic lower-back pain.[13] Another SNRI, milnacipran (Savella) is prescribed for fibromyalgia pain.

Selective serotonin reuptake inhibitors (SSRIs) are the most commonly prescribed antidepressants and are partially effective for diabetic neuropathy, but not to the extent of TCAs. Taken alone, paroxetine (Paxil), escitalopram (Lexapro), sertraline (Zoloft), and fluoxetine (Prozac) have no effect on pain. They do, however, have the potential to boost the analgesic effects of some tricyclic antidepressants. SSRIs can cause agitation, insomnia, gastrointestinal irritation, and erectile dysfunction. Once you start taking these medications, you should never suddenly stop taking them; they must be gradually reduced according to your doctor's instructions.

Anticonvulsants

Drugs that calm the nerves to prevent epileptic seizures are also particularly effective for neuropathic pain. We do not fully understand how anticonvulsants relieve pain, but they are well tolerated in the long term, and nonaddictive.

Gabapentin (Neurontin) is FDA-approved for treating postherpetic neuralgia. It is also widely used to treat sciatica, CRPS, and other neuropathic pain syndromes. Treatment usually begins with moderate doses that are gradually increased until benefit is achieved or until the patient becomes intolerant of the medication's sedating qualities. Gabapentin is well tolerated with few side effects when the dose is gradually increased.

Phenytoin (Dilantin) has been used since 1939 for epilepsy, yet its analgesic properties are not well studied. Usually well tolerated, it is used for neuropathic pain syndromes, particularly trigeminal neuralgia, a type of sharp, stabbing facial nerve pain. Side effects, which may include decreased coordination, shaky hands, slurred speech, and memory problems, often resolve on their own within a few days of starting the medication. Regular blood testing is necessary when this drug is taken.

Carbamazepine (Tegretol, Carbatrol), a drug used for seizures and bipolar disorder, works well for diabetic neuropathy, postherpetic neuralgia, and trigeminal neuralgia. Structurally, carbamazepine is similar to a TCA. Regular blood testing is necessary when this drug is used.

Oxcarbazepine (Trileptal) is a newer antiseizure formulation that is used off-label for diabetic neuropathy and trigeminal neuralgia. Adverse effects reported most commonly include dizziness, sleepiness, and confusion.

Valproic acid (Depakote ER, Depakene, Stavzor) is an anticonvulsant that is also used to treat migraine pain. It can inhibit clotting and may exaggerate the effects of NSAIDs, warfarin (Coumadin), heparin (Plavix), and other blood-thinning medications. Dizziness, indigestion, diarrhea, nausea (when taken without food), skin rashes, and itching are the most common side effects. More serious but less common are liver injury, pancreatitis, and abnormal bleeding.

Clonazepam (Klonopin, Rivotril) may help relieve symptoms of phantom-limb pain and other neuropathic pain.

Topiramate (Topamax) works well for migraine headaches. It causes weight loss, providing a bonus for patients who are overweight or obese. Most side effects, including tingling and fatigue, are well tolerated.

Pregabalin (Lyrica) is FDA-approved for treating the pain of fibromyalgia, diabetic neuropathy, postherpetic neuralgia, and pain resulting from spinal cord injuries. It is believed to reduce pain sensitivity by limiting the release of substance P and glutamate. Pregabalin may cause dizziness; fatigue; problems with vision, concentration, and memory; and loss of balance.

Anesthetics

Numbing agents block nerves that conduct pain signals. Lidocaine or a different local anesthetic can be injected near nerves to temporarily relieve pain or relax cramped or knotted muscles. Postherpetic neuralgia patients generally tolerate a lidocaine patch (Lidoderm) for 12-hour increments without problems. Administered intravenously over hours to days, lidocaine may significantly reduce chronic neuropathic pain for several weeks to a few months. Side effects are usually minimal: mild nausea, drowsiness, and a metallic taste in the mouth are common. Uneven heartbeat, blurred vision, tremors, and other serious complications may develop in people who take beta-blockers, antiarrhythmics (medications to even an erratic heartbeat), or have exposure to other local anesthetics.

NMDA-Receptor Antagonists

Glutamate is an important neurotransmitter that contributes to memory and learning, but it also has a dark side: it activates and overexcites NMDA receptors, contributing to neuropathic pain and hyperalgesia. NMDA antagonists, including methadone, offer alternative treatment for opioid-resistant and neuropathic pain. These formulations disrupt pain messages by blocking NMDA receptors without obstructing other receptors that bind to glutamate. Another NMDA-receptor antagonist, ketamine hydrochloride, has been used as a surgical anesthetic for years but only recently has been considered as treatment for some chronic pain conditions. There has been no long-term scrutiny of ketamine as an analgesic, but a review of clinical data from 1996 through 2002 showed that it satisfactorily reduced phantom-limb pain and postherpetic neuralgia but was ineffective for fibromyalgia and CRPS.[14] Despite these findings, there are many reports of CRPS patients who feel markedly improved after one or more ketamine infusions, including evidence that infusions given over five days relieved severe CRPS pain by 60 percent and that the relief lasted six to 12 weeks.[15] Ketamine may be particularly beneficial as an auxiliary analgesic for patients who need large doses of opioids or have developed opioid tolerance. At low doses, ketamine has a good safety profile with minimal psychological effects (hallucinations and feelings of dissociation) that occur only occasionally. Ketamine can cause dizziness, lightheadedness, and nausea. Repeated use has been associated with liver damage and impaired memory.

Capsaicin is the purified extract of chili peppers, the ingredient that gives them their heat. Rubbed into the skin, capsaicin cream initially burns and then numbs neuralgic pain emanating from nerve endings beneath the surface of the skin. Some patients find that capsaicin temporarily soothes rheumatoid arthritis, osteoarthritis, shingles, fibromyalgia, headaches, and diabetic neuropathy. The only known side effect is possible skin irritation and burning in the eyes and other sensitive areas if they are touched before capsaicin is washed from the hands.

Amantadine and memantine have shown mixed results. Amantadine is used primarily to treat Parkinson's disease and influenza. Long used as a veterinary analgesic, it is being considered as a viable treatment for postherpetic neuralgia, diabetic neuropathy, fibromyalgia, and phantom-limb pain. Memantine works quickly and has few side effects; however, it may work no better than a placebo.[16]

Tramadol (Ultram) is an intriguing medication that does not fit neatly into any analgesic category. Unlike NSAIDs, it has no anti-inflammatory properties. It is not a true opioid, but it binds to mu receptors and acts like a mild opioid agonist. Immediate-release and sustained-release versions of tramadol may soothe a variety of pains. We do not completely understand how tramadol works, but it is believed to attack pain by preventing reuptake of serotonin and norepinephrine and dulling the brain's perception of pain. Side effects are usually minimal and can include nausea, drowsiness, and headache. Seizures are a risk of combining tramadol and some antidepressants.

Other Analgesics for Chronic Pain

Corticosteroids

Prednisone, hydrocortisone, dexamethasone, and other corticosteroids are powerful, quick-acting anti-inflammatories that also relieve pain. (Corticosteroids mimic naturally occurring substances in the body; they are related to but not the same as the steroids that enhance athletic performance.) Moderate doses of corticosteroids (such as prednisone and prednisolone) are most often used as spot relief for flares of pain related to rheumatoid arthritis or to disrupt the pain cycle of CRPS. Injections (methylprednisolone [Solu-Medrol or Depo-Medrol], triamcinolone [Kenalog], and others) given at the point of pain reduce inflammation, especially for bulging discs or disc herniation. Steroid injections can comfort sciatic pain and disc herniation—the effect may last from weeks to years. Injections can also be directed into a troublesome facet joint, but they are not as successful for widespread degenerative or arthritic problems in the spine. Spinal corticosteroid injections are more effective when they are guided with fluoroscopy, a technique that uses an x-ray to guide the needle directly to the painful joints or nerves. Corticosteroids must be used cautiously because of numerous side effects. Limited use rarely causes complications, but long-term use of oral steroids can cause ulcers and bone damage. Because they also raise blood pressure and blood sugar, lower doses are prescribed for diabetics.

Intravenous Immunoglobulin

Produced from donor blood, intravenous immunoglobulin (IVIG) replaces protective antibodies in people who cannot produce them on their own. IVIG is another example of a medication that was accidentally discovered to have analgesic properties. Scientists at Liverpool University showed that low doses of IVIG substantially reduced chronic pain associated with advanced CRPS for an average of five weeks with few side effects (the study was quite small, and the authors noted that it may have been limited by recruitment bias). Almost half of the participants experienced relief; others did not.[17] CRPS is not well understood, but this investigation hints that it is perhaps an autoimmune-induced inflammation in the body, a hypothesis that is supported by other evidence suggesting that people with chronic CRPS tend to have more immune disorders than other people. IVIG neutralizes harmful antibodies produced by a misguided immune system and blocks the autoimmune response of rheumatoid arthritis. Perhaps it acts in a similar way with CRPS.

Beta Blockers and Calcium Channel Blockers

Numerous medications that dilate the blood vessels to lower blood pressure, stabilize irregular heartbeat, and control angina (chest pain) are also used to treat chronic neuropathy. Beta blockers, including propranolol (Inderal), metoprolol succinate (Toprol), and others that lower blood pressure and slow the heart rate by blocking adrenaline are also used to prevent migraines. Medications of this type block the effects of adrenaline and noradrenaline neurotransmitters. Calcium channel blockers, including verapamil (Calan, Verelan, Covera-HS) improve blood flow by decreasing calcium levels in blood vessels and the heart. Neural type (N-type) calcium channel blockers also inhibit pain signals when concentrations of calcium in spinal neurons fire off pain signals to the brain. Ziconotide (Prialt), a synthetic equivalent of a protein from the neurotoxic venom of the ocean cone snail, is an intriguing new drug in this class. It is an N-type calcium channel blocker, and it seems to reduce the nerve-to-nerve progression of pain messages. Ziconotide boosts the effectiveness of opioids and can be useful for a variety of severe pain problems that do not respond to other therapies. A spinal pump must be implanted to deliver the medication directly into the spinal cord. Ziconotide must be used cautiously and judiciously, since it can cause sedation, anxiety, disorientation, and hallucinations.

Muscle Relaxants

Medications that work in the central nervous system to loosen tight muscles and stop spasms temporarily alleviate the pain of fibromyalgia, tension-type headaches, and back conditions. They cause drowsiness, which may be inconvenient for some persons but can be a somewhat welcome side effect for others who are overly anxious and have difficulty sleeping. Muscle relaxants can have side effects of nausea, vomiting, and impaired cognition. Newer data suggest that these side effects supersede the benefit for individuals with chronic arthritis.[18]

Medical Marijuana

Proponents and opponents of medical marijuana cite studies to support their respective positions on the matter. Amid substantial anecdotal evidence from patients, a growing body of research supports the analgesic properties of cannabis extracts. Dronabinol (Marinol), a synthetic form of tetrahydrocannabinol (THC, marijuana's primary active ingredient) is FDA-approved for treating nausea associated with chemotherapy and stimulating the appetites of persons who have AIDS. A small project at Harvard Medical School found that dronabinol used with opioids significantly reduced chronic pain.[19] Among 50 people with HIV and neuropathic pain who smoked marijuana cigarettes three times a day for five days, pain levels were reduced twice as effectively as with a placebo. Similar results have been identified for people with spinal cord injuries, nerve pain, CRPS, and pain related to multiple sclerosis.[20] Despite the seemingly promising potential of these studies, data from large, well-controlled studies are sparse, and not all the findings have been positive. Some studies have found no analgesic effect from THC; at least one effort concluded that it actually increased sensitivity to pain.[21] Most of these studies were small and conducted under less than optimum clinical conditions, yet the Institute of Medicine found enough evidence to conclude that cannabinoids provide mild to moderate pain relief similar to the effect of codeine.

Although several states allow medical marijuana with a doctor's recommendation, the U.S. government classifies marijuana in any form as a schedule I drug, meaning it has a high potential for abuse and no practical medical use. Medical marijuana remains controversial and federally illegal, and it is much in need of well-designed, long-term clinical studies that establish its potential formulation and delivery as an analgesic for chronic pain.

SUMMARY POINTS
- All medications have benefits and risks.
- Medications should be taken at the lowest dose that brings relief and should be taken no longer than necessary.
- Opioids are the mainstay analgesic for acute pain. Their utility is less clear for chronic pain.
- Some patients require pain medications for the rest of their lives.

4

Mind-over-Pain Therapies

Aristotle was on the right track when he said that pain is an emotion. Although pain signals are purely physical, the brain, with its massively complex reaction, determines how the pain experience unfolds. It is not entirely accurate to say that pain is "all in the head," yet it is a true mind-body phenomenon with two interwoven elements: the neural signal and the emotional response. Treatment involves manipulation of one or the other or both. We use medications and physical interventions to partially or totally block pain signals and therapeutic techniques to retrain the mind's reaction to pain. In the best scenario, engaging the mind limits the need for medication or eliminates it altogether. Although much of the brain's workings remains mysterious, flexing your emotional muscles can either increase your pain and affect your overall health negatively or act as the most powerful pain reliever known.

Pain begins as a physical reaction to a stimulus, but its interpretation by the mind is cloaked with an individual's feelings, experiences, and expectations. Your past and present emotional state has everything to do with how you feel pain and deal with it. Resisting pain is instinctive, a subconscious and automatic action that serves pain more than it serves the person. While fear, anxiety, depression, and other harmful emotions heighten pain perception, reframing these thoughts can greatly modify that perception so that pain becomes less intense and demands less attention. Leveraging mind-body techniques may not eliminate pain, but it will strengthen your ability to cope. In this way, pain becomes a motivator rather than a detractor from the things you want in life, despite the discomfort your body may experience. Replacing harmful thoughts takes conscious effort, but the benefits can be life-changing.

People faced with extraordinary circumstances often temporarily override pain signals through conscious effort or distraction: wounded soldiers may feel no pain until they leave the battlefield, and injured athletes are often unaware of a painful injury until the game ends. You do not need to face a life-threatening situation to experience the same benefit. With a bit of practice, you can harness the same mindful power to triumph over your pain.

How Emotional Stress Heightens Pain

Feelings shape reactions to virtually everything we experience in life. Body, thoughts, and emotions function in concert to shape our awareness. We react positively to humor, kindness, and things that make us feel good, but it is human nature to move away from life experiences that are emotionally or physically uncomfortable, rather than trying to understand or embrace them. When pain develops, the brain integrates the physical sensation with thoughts, memories, expectations, and other emotional and psychological factors. Our individual emotional baggage affects how we process and feel pain, forming unique personal perceptions and responses.

How do you respond when pain never really goes away? Thinking "I just can't take this anymore" or "This horrible pain keeps me from playing with my children" tells your mind that you are helpless against your pain. When you habitually think this way, whether consciously or subconsciously, you give your mind marching orders to maintain the painful status quo. You will never find relief from the anger, frustration, and sadness you feel as long as your mind works to make your negative thinking a reality. Pessimistic or cynical feelings about tenacious pain make coping more difficult, contributing to a recipe for continued misery. Frustration when arthritis robs you of the ability to open a jar or tie your shoes. Anger because you can no longer work. Fear that your pain will just get worse. Depression because you cannot envision a future without pain. These tension-producing thoughts intensify pain and create greater unhappiness, dysfunction, and disability (table 4.1).

TABLE 4.1   Impacts of negative emotional factors

Emotional factors that increase pain	
Anger	Depression
Anguish	Disappointment
Anxiety	Fear
Bitterness	Helplessness
Cynicism	Hopelessness

Other impacts of negative emotional factors	
Difficulty concentrating	Frustration
Disability	Irritability
Dysfunction	Loss of control
Fatigue	Narrowed view of life

The brain does not differentiate between emotional and physical pain; either type stimulates the same areas. It simply recognizes and responds to pain as pain, regardless of the source. Deep-rooted adverse emotions sabotage well-being in other ways as well, sapping energy and inhibiting motivation to self-manage pain. They also create neurochemical changes in the body that decrease pain resistance, perpetuating the cycle of pain that leads to more harmful emotions.

Preoccupation with the negative aspects of a particular circumstance, especially pain, can be particularly harmful. It may seem counterintuitive to think of pain in any other way, but *catastrophizing*—thinking "This pain will only get worse," "Pain is ruining my life," or similar thoughts— actually increases pain sensitivity. Catastrophizing creates a negative mind-set that shifts focus away from what is real, causing you to dwell instead on the worst possible outcome. The tendency to catastrophize during pain, which is more common among women than men, elevates anxiety and worry, amplifying the pain experience and emotional distress. Catastrophizing is a greater predictor of decreased quality of life than pain intensity alone is.[1]

Confronting Depression and Anxiety

Pain that does not go away can be a dejecting burden that delays recovery and intensifies suffering. Experts estimate that up to 80 percent of

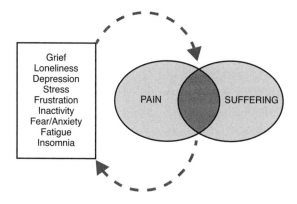

Grief
Loneliness
Depression
Stress
Frustration
Inactivity
Fear/Anxiety
Fatigue
Insomnia

PAIN   SUFFERING

FIGURE 4.1. Persistent pain can create a cycle of emotional and psychological issues that makes pain worse.

individuals who have chronic pain suffer from depression, and many also have anxiety disorders. This is not surprising, given the extreme limitations chronic pain often imposes on life. Over time, constant negative emotions become ingrained in your brain; it can be difficult to encourage more positive emotions that you may have abandoned since your pain began. Overlapping pain and depression form a vicious cycle: sustained pain alters your mood, and unresolved emotions cause pain (figure 4.1). The more you hurt, the lower your pain threshold becomes, and this repeated sequence further deepens depression. But we have tools to disrupt the cycle. We use analgesics and antidepressants that restrict chemical messages in the brain to affect both conditions. Psychological counseling, stress-reduction techniques, and physical activity can also help.

. . . .

I hurt my back at the age of 23 while working as a nursing assistant. At the time, I couldn't fathom how it would change my life forever. Ten years and two spinal fusions later, I suffer from debilitating chronic pain—all day, every day. It's the first sensation I feel when I open my eyes and the last thing I feel as I go to sleep. Living with suffocating pain while the world around you is oblivious and unconcerned can be so lonely it's chilling. It has challenged me mentally and physically in more ways than I could ever imagine.

Suffering can easily cause depression that spirals downward into paralyzing self-loathing. It's easy to think that you want to stop living. As I fought to transcend the darkest time of my life, I knew that I was sick; sicker than I had ever been. I kept telling myself to just "snap out of it," or "get over it," but I couldn't. Day after day I sunk deeper and deeper into a swamp of the monumental depression that entrapped me. I was in a catatonic state; I suffered extreme memory loss and was unable to process the most basic information. I was emotionally unstable, anxious, impatient, angry, and cried excessively.

Finally I turned to Dr. Richeimer for help. If he'd given me a prescription for an antidepressant and sent me on my way, I probably would've had a nervous breakdown by now. Instead, I am a success story because he and his patient-attentive team took a holistic approach to my recovery that was nothing short of miraculous. My team—Dr. Richeimer and a physical therapist, an occupational therapist, and a psychiatrist—treated me as a whole person. They cared enough to not just get me through my immediate crisis, but to help me prevent myself from ever falling into such a deep depression again; that included having the tools I needed to deal with stress and learn how to pace myself physically and emotionally when I returned to work. These tools helped me pull myself through the crisis and provided me with knowledge to foster prevention. That is why I am stronger and happier today than ever before.

Making the decision to live in positivity and having a support system is essential to surviving chronic pain. I am blessed with an amazing family, and my rewarding career as a nurse enables me to deflect my energies and turn something very ugly into something beautiful. Throughout this journey I have learned that I want to live my life joyfully, and to do this I must lean on my support systems and not allow this crippling disease to steal any more precious time from me. For me, living in a state of depression is not an option!

—Danielle

. . . .

Change Your Thinking, Change Your Life

You can change the way you feel by overhauling the way you think about your pain. If you believe your pain will become worse, it will. Believe instead that it will not control your life, and replace thoughts of despair with visions of how you would like your life to be, and you will feel better. This is more than fantasy. It is evidence-based fact. Reframing your thoughts to think about pain in a less judgmental way redirects your mind to experience pain differently and to release pain-inhibiting signals along descending pain pathways.[2] Learning to let go of unhealthy feelings and replace them with healthy self-talk ("I can control how much attention I give my pain" and "Some things I cannot do, but there is much that I can do") counteracts harmful alterations that chronic pain makes to the mind and body and creates a more meaningful and positive existence. Launching a daily barrage of positive affirmative thoughts may not bring about the cure you hope for, but it will shift pain from being the dominant force in your life.

An experienced psychiatrist or psychologist can help you sort out these issues; that recommendation often makes a person balk at the implication of needing a "head" doctor—"I'm not crazy and I don't need my head examined!" However, psychotherapy is an important cornerstone of any multidisciplinary approach to relieving pervasive pain. In pain management, psychotherapy is just as useful for people who are psychologically healthy as for those who are not. Psychotherapy also helps you deal with anxiety or concerns that arise when loved ones underestimate your pain or do not believe it is real.

. . . .

In 1997, I thought I had dislocated my left shoulder when I fell from a loading dock, but I found out it was more serious—I had a massive tear in my rotator cuff. My first surgery didn't go well; it only made the pain worse. My doctor told me that my tendons were also torn. After 10 surgeries my shoulder still didn't feel right, and at that point, he told me that it was chronic pain that could not be repaired and nothing else could be done. I was very, very depressed. I didn't want to accept that I would always have such pain, so I saw another doctor who performed an acromioplasty that shaved bone to relieve pressure on the rotator cuff. When that didn't work, he moved a muscle from my back to my shoulder, but that also failed. Then I had screws implanted to hold my shoulder together—more surgery—but while in the hospital, I developed a serious infection. I remained there for an entire month. My last shoulder surgery fused the bone, but after that I still had more pain than I could manage and my depression got worse. My doctors prescribed lots of different medications, including antidepressants and acetaminophen combined with hydrocodone. I had other procedures as well: a stellate ganglion injection to try to block the pain (that didn't work) and another minor surgery to implant a spinal cord stimulator. The stimulator has helped, but I still take methadone for pain. I have bad days when I am severely depressed and have to call my clinical psychologist.

—Jessie

. . . .

. . . .

I underwent a circumcision as an adult. Unfortunately an infection occurred and the sutured area did not heal properly, resulting in the development of scar tissue. Although the infection healed, it left an abscess in the soft tissue in the shaft of my penis. Whenever I sat, the scar tissue caused friction against other nearby soft tissue; the best analogy to describe it is geologic tectonic plates that rub against each other resulting in an earthquake. I have a very high tolerance for pain, but this was excruciating. It felt as though a thousand tiny knives were stabbing my private parts. My entire musculoskeletal system tensed because the nerve pain was so great, causing headaches that felt like a python had wrapped itself around my neck. My head felt as though it would explode. Commuting and sitting at work were terrible experiences that I just had to endure. The only relief was when I was standing or lying down. My general practitioner prescribed gabapentin, but it made me sluggish and sleepy. I fell into a deep depression, and for two and a half years not a day went by that I did not consider ending my life.

When I was referred to the pain center at the University of Southern California, my life not only changed, it was saved. The duloxetine (Cymbalta) that Dr. Richeimer prescribed helped, and my employer provided an adjustable workstation that allowed me to stand whenever I was in pain. With the medication and the sit/stand workstation, I had less pain, and as a result, the muscles in my back, neck, and shoulders that caused my headaches relaxed. At the same time, psychological and physical therapies helped my recovery. When Dr. Richeimer suggested that I see a psychologist, I didn't think it was necessary; in hindsight, however, I am very grateful for his recommendation. I needed someone to talk to, and my psychologist made me become accountable for certain beneficial action items. She is a big part of my recovery. Prior to the circumcision, I was physically active, but after the procedure, I was in too much pain to exercise. My psychologist and physical therapist pushed me to become physically active again, which cleared up my mind. The duloxetine *deadened some of the nerve pain and I was able to get back to swimming, yoga, and walking.*

—Lawrence

....

Altering Your Expectations

Your expectations of pain have a significant role in determining your experience. Anticipating that your pain will magically vanish is improbable and unrealistic, and believing that you cannot control it leads to acute stress, which only causes more pain. If you feel powerless and alone with your pain, and you believe it can get no better, it won't get better. Assume instead that your pain may remain to some degree but will not impede your happiness, and that your life will improve. Training yourself to think positively about your pain—you did not give this condition to yourself, but you do have the power to make the best of your life—is intrinsic to pain management. Focus on the areas where you have control, rather than where you do not, and you can change how you react.

Your brain's pain network responds to your expectation of how well medication will work.[3] Positive expectations reduce pain perception (the placebo affect); negative expectations (the *nocebo effect*) amplify it.[4] With an open mind and proactive thinking, you can transform your thinking

DIFFERENTIATING BETWEEN PSYCHIATRISTS AND PSYCHOLOGISTS

Although both psychiatrists and psychologists engage in psychotherapy, their training and services differ. Psychiatrists are physicians who have spent at least three years in a mental health residency after medical school. Psychologists, who have either a Ph.D. (Doctor of Philosophy) or a Psy.D. (Doctor of Psychology) degree, have received graduate training in clinical or counseling psychology. Unlike psychiatrists, they do not attend medical school, and in most states they do not have prescribing privileges. Psychiatrists provide comprehensive medically based evaluations and diagnoses, medications, and talking therapy, while psychologists provide evaluations and treatment through talk-based therapy.

into a pain-management tool. If you feel a sense of dread and dependency each time you swallow your daily pain medication, why not change your thinking to transform that negative experience into a ritual with positive effect? As you swallow your medication, imagine it flooding your body with comfort and relief. Close your eyes and visualize the pills, capsules, or liquid rushing through your bloodstream and overwhelming your source of pain with a brilliant healing force that allows you to be more functional throughout the day or rest more peacefully during the night. Do not just go through the motions. The more vividly you can imagine this, the better.

The brain has the ability to turn pain on or off. In a well-documented study, researchers trained monkeys to press a lever in response to a light. The lever triggered a brief painful heat stimulus, and as expected, the monkeys' nerves then fired (electrodes implanted in their spinal cords recorded the activity) and they quickly pulled their hands away. After repeating this exercise daily for several days, researchers noted exactly the same results—the monkeys' pain neurons fired after the light, even when the heat was not administered.[5] Similar conditioning also occurs in humans. In their anticipation of pain, patients who have repetitive injections often say "ouch" when their skin is swabbed with alcohol, before the needle punctures their skin. Functional MRI scans of people's brains show that the cingulate cortex is activated in the same way whether pain is anticipated or actually felt.[6]

. . . .

Before seeing a therapist, my attention was constantly focused on why my pain didn't go away. Every morning when I awoke without the benefit of my dreamed-of magical cure, my first thoughts were "How much pain do I have today?" and "What will I have to give up because of it?" Every day I lived in a cycle of anger and despair. Once I realized how damaging my thinking really was and how it only made the pain worse, I changed my mind-set from needing to be pain-free to being happy even though I had some pain, and I began to do much better.

—Angela

. . . .

Mindful Meditation

Contrary to what many people think, you do not need to stand on your head or twist your body like a pretzel to meditate. Nor do you need to practice for years to enjoy a fruitful practice of meditation. Meditation, the reflective practice of quieting one's mind, has been practiced in one form or another for thousands of years. Often described as the space between thoughts, meditation self-regulates attention to still the mind and body, and it channels perception toward a positive direction. It is recognized and valued as a relaxation tool that is practiced by people in all walks of life. The most common form of meditation practiced in the West is *mindfulness,* being aware and attentive to the present. When you're mindful, you observe your thoughts and feelings without judging them as good or bad, beneficial or harmful. You allow your mind to be fluid, to flow from one thought to the next without focusing on anything specific, including pain. Being mindful of the present prevents the anticipation of pain. Routinely practicing mindfulness improves people's quality of life related to many painful disorders, including chronic low-back pain, arthritis, and irritable bowel syndrome.[7]

Mindfulness is good medicine. It quiets the body as it relaxes the mind, so that people become less fearful of their pain. Mindful meditation is a potent way to rid the body of tension that occurs as a natural reaction to pain. Accepting pain rather than fighting it is a difficult concept for Western minds to understand and embrace, yet doing so is an important step in self-managing pain. With practice, patients become adept at observing their pain without reacting to it, providing a measure of control whenever pain occurs. Thus, they can focus on other, more positive aspects of life. Regularly practicing mindfulness also affords the brain time to rest, rejuvenate, and recover from the pressures and strain of constant thought. Mastering the technique, however, takes some effort to move beyond our normal tendency to allow random, unfocused thoughts (table 4.2).

TABLE 4.2 Five myths about meditation

Myth	Fact
Meditation is just a fad	Meditation has been practiced for thousands of years
Meditation is an escape from reality	Meditation increases awareness
Meditation requires years of practice	Skills grow over time and with practice, but benefits can be realized almost immediately
Meditation is practical only for yogis	Anyone can benefit
Meditation is a state of bliss without thought	Meditation creates awareness of thoughts so that they can be directed at will

Other Types of Meditation

Mindfulness is the core of Buddhism and the foundation for various types of meditation, but many different types of meditative practices also encourage mental clarity:

- Mantra meditation involves repetitive chanting of a word or phrase.
- Focused meditation strives to maintain concentration on a single sound, mantra, or thought.
- Movement meditation includes swaying, undulating, or dancing with or without music as it focuses attention.
- Spiritual meditation aims for concentration on a particular soulful dilemma or question in an effort to connect with a higher power.

Cognitive Behavioral Techniques

Cognitive behavior therapy (CBT) is the core of many psychologically therapeutic regimens. It is usually a short-term treatment for anxiety, eating issues, addiction, or other specific problems, including chronically painful conditions. Based on the theory that our feelings and behaviors are caused by what we think rather than by external influences, CBT helps patients to acknowledge discouraging thoughts that occur with or without their knowledge. Participating in individual or group sessions, patients learn how to replace habitually harmful thought pat-

TABLE 4.3   Reframing negative thoughts about pain

Harmful thoughts	Beneficial thoughts
I just can't take it	I can relax to feel better
It will never go away	It waxes and wanes
It will only get worse	I can control how much attention I give it
It will ruin my life	My life can still be full of purpose and meaning
I have nothing to look forward to but pain	I cannot do certain things, but there is much I can do
I will never be happy again	My body is in pain, but I control my mind, and there I can be happy

terns with supportive affirmations that shift consciousness away from an obsession with pain. (An individual's expectations of how successfully CBT will affect her pain can also affect treatment outcome, another example of the brain's influence.)[8] By changing the way we think, we change the way we feel, even when our circumstances remain the same (table 4.3).

Hypnosis

Clinical hypnosis is not the same as an entertainer putting someone under a spell so the person will cluck like a chicken whenever he hears a code word. Conducted by a qualified hypnotherapist, hypnosis can decrease one's sensitivity to severe or ceaseless pain, depending on the individual's susceptibility to hypnotic suggestion—most people are moderately receptive, while some are resistant. A significant body of research attests to the effectiveness of hypnosis for chronic pain conditions such as fibromyalgia and irritable bowel syndrome.[9] An analysis of 13 studies of hypnosis used for chronic pain (studies involving headaches were excluded) indicates that hypnotic intervention produces meaningful reductions in perceived pain. In some patients, that perception lasted for several months. (The authors of the analysis noted that more sophisticated research with larger sample sizes and more rigorous controls is needed.)[10]

Hypnosis is no hocus-pocus. It is a state of intense concentration that allows patients to focus on the resolution of a specific problem; it's similar to being so absorbed in a book or movie that you become unaware of everything else. Hypnosis tunes out the conscious mind so that the subconscious becomes more active. Persons in a hypnotic state are comfortable, relaxed, and fully awake. They are also open to suggestion, which is advantageous for separating destructive memories of pain from expectations and replacing unhealthy thoughts with beneficial ideas. People usually need 4 to 10 one-hour sessions before they experience less pain. Therapists usually teach their patients to induce self-hypnosis as needed.

Guided Imagery

Have you ever awakened with the memory of a particular dream and wondered how your brain could conjure up such fantastical or bizarre thoughts? You can turn that capability to your advantage against pain with *guided imagery,* a type of self-induced hypnotic state triggered by the use of mental images to achieve deep relaxation. The goal is to tune out distractions as much as possible. You control your breathing, relax your muscles, and concentrate on positive thoughts and images. Your brain picks up these cues and takes over.

A guided-imagery session begins by getting into a relaxed state that allows you to mentally travel and use imagery to control your pain. Some people visualize going to the beach and floating on water that absorbs all

> ### PSYCHONEUROIMMUNOLOGY
>
> *Psychoneuroimmunology* is the study of the interdependence between brain and body, the interactions between the nervous system, the immune system, and thought. The basis for psychoneuroimmunology is the understanding that the same bodily chemicals that operate our bodies also influence our emotions. Scientific evidence supports the premise that the mind and the body are fully intertwined, bridged by emotions and feelings; what we think and feel directly impacts our health and well-being.

pain and tension. Others imagine a visit to the brain's control center, where they turn knobs and switches to dial down their pain. Some use their imaginations to converse with wizards who use magic wands to banish pain. Individuals who are in pain sometimes form a mental picture of inhaling a healing breath or vapor of a certain color; when they exhale, the color is different, reflecting the absence of pain and tension. With guided imagery, nothing is too far-fetched. The more vivid the imagery, the better. Some people have wildly imaginative experiences from the start. Others develop more creative visualizations as they become comfortable with techniques of the practice. Anyone, even those who doubt their ability to create helpful mental images, can learn to use guided imagery. Visualization is beneficial when it is affirmative. But beware of less-than-positive imagery. Painting a more painful picture of your future sows harmful negative images in the mind.

Positive Psychology

Many branches of psychology involve a focus on depression, dysfunction, and other negative aspects of the human psyche. *Positive psychology,* a newer complementary therapy, emphasizes the opposite, focusing on aspects that make life worth living. This school of thought is a broad evidence-based study of the emotions and experiences that affect happiness. The pioneer of this fast-growing field is Dr. Martin Seligman, director of the Positive Psychology Center at the University of Pennsylvania and the author of several books on the subject, including *Flourish: A Visionary New Understanding of Happiness* and *Well-Being, Learned Optimism:*

How to Change Your Mind and Your Life. Seligman's goal is to improve the quality of life by dwelling on what is right rather than focusing on what is wrong and to help people flourish by building strength rather than patching weakness. Positive psychology is an effort to better understand and maximize human happiness, a much-needed prescription for individuals who live with chronic pain. People who practice positive psychology immerse themselves in activities and actions that advance creativity, achievement, joy, and other emotional strengths that build contentment and resilience.

Stress Management and Relaxation Tools

Stress has always been a part of life and remains so today, despite our achievements and modern conveniences. We struggle with family and work issues, cope with traffic jams and the rising cost of living, and try to manage medical bills. Add pain into the mix, and you have a recipe for even greater stress and the collateral damage it causes. Whether it is physical or psychological in nature, stress affects pain in the same way— it interferes with the brain's ability to filter pain signals. Stress and anxiety also raise blood pressure, create fatigue, contribute to depression, and cause a host of mind-body ailments. Both reactions increase pain by stimulating the sympathetic nervous system to provoke the *fight-or-flight response,* a biochemical defense mechanism left over from our hunter-gatherer days. Faced with a possibly life-threatening situation, our cavemen ancestors experienced a rush of adrenaline that increased their heart rate and respiration to prepare their bodies to fight or flee. Unlike those ancestors, most of us need not worry about being attacked by predators, but many aspects of modern life are disturbing, and we retain the same response to stressful situations whether they are real or only perceived.

Unless you act to rid yourself of constant stress and anxiety, your muscles remain tensed and your body acts as though it is in a constant state of danger, secreting neurochemicals that intensify pain. Relaxation decreases cortisol, the so-called "stress hormone" that suppresses the immune system, raises blood pressure, and decreases cognitive performance. Relaxing calms the mind and counteracts these harmful changes.

Managing stress is important for everyone; it is especially critical for people with chronic pain, because it helps to overcome the negative impacts of overlapping stress and pain.

When the mind is relaxed, we can focus on other thoughts that distract the brain from sensing painful sensations. Taking steps to actively reduce stress can help in these ways:

- ease tense muscles that magnify pain
- improve your ability to cope with pain
- reduce the tendency to catastrophize
- relieve frustration about the limitations pain puts on your life
- reduce mental and physical fatigue caused by fighting persistent pain
- increase concentration

Biofeedback

You may not be familiar with *biofeedback,* even though you use the same principle every time you step on a scale or check your temperature with a thermometer. Biofeedback is just another way of providing information about what is going on in your body. It is a credible tool for relieving anxiety, depression, high blood pressure, and urinary incontinence. Given the role of stress in chronic pain, the potential for biofeedback as a self-management tool is probably much broader than we know. It is frequently used to manage back pain and headaches, including migraines. More research is needed to determine whether it might also work well against other types of pain.

Using monitoring instruments that emit a beep or display a light as the patient becomes more relaxed, biofeedback trains people to modulate involuntary bodily processes with deep breathing and other relaxation techniques. By watching a visual display of skin temperature, muscle tension, pulse, or heart rate, people can readily see how their own actions affect these processes. In time, they learn to sense and control these physiological processes without the instruments, voluntarily producing a relaxation response whenever pain becomes too strong or intrusive.

Therapists use several biofeedback therapies. (Most professionals who provide biofeedback specialize in certain disorders, so it is worthwhile to find someone who has experience treating your specific pain condition.) *Thermal biofeedback* (also called *temperature biofeedback*) measures skin temperature. A sensor attached to the patient's finger sends signals to the biofeedback monitor, which reflects the temperature of the hand; the foot is sometimes used instead. Stress causes a noticeable drop in hand temperature as the fight-or-flight response redirects blood flow to the brain and large muscles. Relaxation reverses this effect. Thermal biofeedback is especially productive for headache sufferers. As people watch the rise and fall of their hand temperature on the biofeedback monitor, they can control their pain by calming their thoughts and relaxing, thereby warming their hands, when they notice a decrease in temperature. *Electromyography* biofeedback measures muscle tension and helps people learn to relax excessively contracted muscle groups. *Electroencephalography* feedback is a more sophisticated process that visually records brain-wave activity.

✸ BIOFEEDBACK FOR MIGRAINE

RON HAD A LONG HISTORY OF MIGRAINE HEADACHES, which frequently sent him to the emergency room. After many years of trying numerous analgesics and beta blockers, his debilitating headaches persisted. Desperate to get his life back on track, Ron was receptive to the comprehensive pain plan we developed for him. He was open to trying different medications, and he didn't mind keeping a pain log to identify food triggers and sources of stress. We recommended that he also consult with a mental health expert. She recommended electromyography and thermal biofeedback. Ron was skeptical; it all sounded too New Age, but he was motivated to get better and agreed to try it.

Ron was nervous when he was first hooked up to the sensors, but his interest peaked as soon as he understood what he was seeing on the monitor. During 16 biofeedback sessions, Ron learned how to consciously isolate, contract, and release muscles in his face, neck, and shoulders. He also saw that his hand temperature was a signpost of his level of tension. The mental image of soaking his hands in warm water effectively relaxed him. Once he became adept with the techniques, he used them twice a day at home to calm and control his migraines. Using biofeedback was not a perfect cure for Ron. It did not eliminate his headaches. Combined with medication, however, biofeedback gave Ron a measure of control over the stress in his life and helped him to reduce the frequency of his headaches by nearly 50 percent. ☼

Deep Breathing

Breathing is one of the body's many involuntary mechanisms; we do not need to think about it to make it happen. But we can consciously control our breath, unlike other involuntary functions. Most of us breathe shallowly, from our upper chest, especially when we are tense or anxious. Breathing deeply from the diaphragm for a few minutes instantly counteracts stressful effects. Practiced anywhere, at home, in a busy office, or stuck in traffic, it expands the lungs, pumping healthy oxygen into the body; the oxygen lowers our blood pressure, slows our heart rate, and relaxes our muscles. Concentrating on the breath, and nothing but the breath, quiets the mind.

Humor

Pain is no laughing matter, but humor has a proven place in positive psychology. Laughter as good medicine is not a new idea. The Old Testament (Proverbs 17:22) advises that "a cheerful heart is good medicine, but a crushed spirit dries up the bones." Humor diverts the mind from pain and dispels tension. Studies reveal that laughing boosts immune cells, releases endorphins, and lowers hormones that contribute to stress and pain. Researchers at the University of Oxford set out to determine

how laughter might benefit people with pain. They measured the pain
thresholds of participants before and after they watched (as a group) 15
minutes of a live comedy show and clips of *Mr. Bean* and *Friends* television shows. Afterward, pain thresholds were about 10 percent better than
before. People who watched the shows alone had only slight improvement, while the control group, who watched nonhumorous videos, experienced no change.[11] A good chuckle or a rollicking belly laugh temporarily releases tension and lightens mood. Have you ever noticed how
quickly kids rebound from sadness or pain? It may have something to
do with laughter, since children laugh more freely and more frequently
than adults.

One dramatic endorsement for laughter as part of a healing regimen
is Norman Cousins's memoir, *Anatomy of an Illness.* A well-known jour-
nalist, editor, and activist, Cousins was also a professor at the University
of California-Los Angeles School of Medicine. His research convinced
him that if negative emotions produce harmful chemical changes in the
body, positive emotions would have the opposite effect. He tested his
theory when he was diagnosed with an unusually severe degenerative
spinal condition. Told that he probably would not survive, Cousins em-
barked on a self-directed recovery plan that included massive doses of
vitamin C supplemented with plenty of upbeat attitude and lots of laughter. Every day he enjoyed television episodes of *Candid Camera,* watched
Marx Brothers comedies, and read lighthearted books that buoyed his
spirits and hope. "I made the joyous discovery that ten minutes of genuine belly laughter had an anesthetic effect and would give me at least two
hours of pain-free sleep," he wrote. "When the painkilling effect of the

laughter wore off, we would switch on the motion picture projector again, and not infrequently, it would lead to another pain-free interval."

Journaling

Committing your innermost thoughts to paper or an electronic document is another cathartic way to deal with adverse emotions. The key to writing as therapy is to let your thoughts flow freely without controlling, censoring, or editing them. Record how you feel about your pain and its effect on your life. What you write may surprise you. But be cautious about the time you spend journaling so that it does not keep you focused on your pain and become counterproductive.

SUMMARY POINTS
- **The mind influences how we experience pain and how we react to it.**
- **Our minds are highly adaptive.**
- **Thinking negatively about pain makes it worse.**
- **Using positive thinking, imagery, and other mind-body techniques can reduce pain and improve coping skills.**

Body-over-Pain Therapies

Along with medication and changing the way one thinks, physical intervention is crucial in an overall pain-management strategy. The treatments described in this chapter relieve pain so that daily life requires less medication or none at all.

Get Moving, Get Better

The stress of persistent pain quickly takes a toll on the body: muscles tighten and become stiff, making even the simplest tasks difficult. Our tendency to stop moving when we hurt is a protective human reflex, but it deconditions muscles and perpetuates pain. The more you hurt, the less you move, and the less you move, the less you are able to accomplish. A sedentary lifestyle increases pain and makes for poor overall health. Regular physical activity, however, works against pain and reduces your risk for heart disease, diabetes, cancer, and many other diseases. A progressive fitness regimen yields impressive benefits for your mind and body, elevating your mood, restoring your functionality, and putting you on a path to a brighter future. A sizable amount of research bears this out. An analysis of 33 different studies concluded that exercise reduces pain and improves physical functionality related to osteoarthritis, rheumatoid arthritis, and fibromyalgia.[1] It produces similar benefits for other painful conditions, including back and neck pain and also chest pain after breast cancer surgery.[2] Even something as simple as walking, which stimulates blood flow and increases endorphins, can help to suppress pain.

Not just any exercise will do. Pursuing even the least demanding movement may seem unfathomable when pain leaves you miserable and fatigued, but movement is good medicine. Although you may not feel the energy or motivation to exercise, the right kind of activity is the very thing that can enhance your pain tolerance and return more functionality to your life. Initially, exercising may be difficult and cause some discomfort, but it should never be so strenuous that it is harmful. Any new exercise program should be undertaken only with the guidance of your doctor or a qualified physical therapist, preferably one who is experienced with your type of pain. Physical therapists are licensed professionals who hold either a Doctor of Physical Therapy (D.P.T.) or a Master of Physical Therapy (M.P.T.) degree. A good physical therapist can guide you through customized movements that do not intensify your pain or cause further harm to already damaged joints and muscles. She can show you how to move in a way that is both safe and beneficial and help you to safely push your physical limits—just enough, but not too much—resulting in more extensive rehabilitation than you might otherwise achieve on your own.

Too much of the wrong activity can make pain worse. If running or jogging are out of the question, you may be able to manage and enjoy cycling, which is easier on painful knees and hips. Aquatic therapy, including aerobics performed in warm water, helps to alleviate inflammation; the buoyancy of the water protects the body from the stress of gravity and from jerky or jarring movements that might otherwise cause pain. No matter which type of exercise you choose, use caution not to move too quickly, stretch or twist too far, or do so much that your pain becomes worse. As you become more comfortable, you may decide to enroll in an exercise class or pursue personal training; inform your instructor or fitness professional of your condition, so he can demonstrate how to move safely and get the most out of your workout.

Exercise improves a person's sleep patterns. Sleep problems often plague individuals who have chronic pain. Worry, depression, or the pain itself diminishes the quantity and quality of your sleep. Some medications also encourage insomnia. Sleeping aids can help, but practicing relaxation and behavioral therapy techniques can help you get more normal sleep without side effects. When restorative sleep patterns improve, pain symptoms usually do, too.[3] Physically active individuals sleep longer and more deeply than those who are sedentary. Exercise also helps to alleviate sleep apnea, a common disruptive sleep disorder that abruptly stops the breath.

. . . .

My pain began in 1982 from a ballet injury. It took nearly 14 years before I was diagnosed with complex regional pain syndrome, known then as reflex sympathetic dystrophy. Since then, I've developed fibromyalgia, chronic fatigue syndrome, irritable bowel syndrome, and osteoarthritis. On a scale of 0 to 10, with 10 being the highest pain imaginable, my pain was almost always a 10. I was bedridden for a decade because of it, unable to speak for five of those years, and rarely got much sleep. I began to improve when I finally switched to a pain-management specialist. Part of my multidisciplinary treatment was getting back to exercise. It's the first thing I do every morning (except Sunday, my day off). I swim nearly a mile three mornings a week, whether or not I have slept or am in pain. If my right arm, which was broken a year ago and is often as painful as my CRPS, gives me too much pain, I kick the laps I can't finish or I swim one-armed laps. On the other three mornings, I do an intense 45-minute ballet-and-Pilates workout, followed by 15 to 20 minutes of Feldenkrais. My morning exercise wakes me up and gets my body and mind ready for a productive day. I feel better when I move. Fifteen years after my pain started, I began seeing a pain psychologist, who taught me to use relaxation and biofeedback. My pain level tapered to between a 5 and a 7, and my body became more relaxed every week. In 2009, I achieved partial CRPS remission. Rarely, my pain now spikes to a 9, but it is generally between levels 2 and 4.

—Cynthia

Passive Physical Therapies

Exercise and movement are examples of active physical therapy. Various passive therapies also temporarily relieve pain. Applying cold (an ice pack or a bag of frozen vegetables wrapped in a towel), heat (a warm bath or a heating pad), or alternating hot and cold to painful areas for 20 minutes temporarily eases painful joints, muscles, tendons, and ligaments. Ultrasound, which generates heat with sound waves, increases circulation to soft tissues and promotes healing. Physical therapists sometimes perform ultrasound treatments just before exercise to make movement easier. (This is not the same as diagnostic ultrasound.) It takes time to break old habits. If your body is accustomed to holding tension, the following therapies can help you become more relaxed.

Therapeutic Massage

If you have never had a massage, you might be surprised at how therapeutic it can be. The healing power of touch soothes muscles and mind. Massage by a licensed massage therapist—preferably someone who deals with pain patients—releases muscle tension and softens connective tissues. Massage has been shown to relieve pain from fibromyalgia, tension-type headaches, back pain, and some types of osteoarthritis. Depending on your condition and level of pain, however, certain forms of massage may be too forceful and even harmful.

Several types of massage are commonly used to relieve pain.

- *Swedish massage* involves kneading or tapping muscles with firm, gentle strokes to increase circulation and theoretically remove toxins. The masseuse may also rapidly move her hands over the body to relax and invigorate.
- *Myofascial release massage* uses long stretching movements to release the *fascia* (the connective tissue surrounding muscles).
- *Trigger-point massage* (also referred to as neuromuscular therapy) applies focused finger pressure directly on specific tight muscle fibers.
- *Deep tissue massage* is similar to classic massage techniques, but it exerts more pressure in slower, more forceful strokes, concentrating on deeper layers of muscle and connective tissue to relieve stiffness.

Rolfing Structural Integration is an intense and often painful manipulation of the fascia or connective tissues between muscle and bone. It was developed by Ida Rolf, a biochemist who believed that bodily pain results from imbalanced alignment that is reinforced by gravity and poor posture. Unlike practitioners of traditional massage, which focuses on the muscles, and chiropractic manipulation, which emphasizes spinal alignment, Rolfing practitioners aggressively use their fists, elbows, and knuckles to "restructure" fascia to release stress, ease pain, and promote correct posture and balance. Research is limited, and there is no evidence that Rolfing treatment relieves pain.

Trager Psychophysical Integration sessions include passive and active components. During table work sessions, a practitioner uses his hands to isolate and gently manipulate joints, muscles, and fascia. These sessions are reinforced by more active "Mentastics," freeform dancelike movements performed at home or in a group setting. These movements are intended to decrease tension by recalling the feeling of deep relaxation. Very little research on this therapy exists. A limited study found that it relieved shoulder pain in patients with spinal cord injury as effectively as acupuncture.[4]

The objective of the *Alexander technique* is somewhat similar to Rolfing: teaching individuals to use their muscles more efficiently to correct habitual postures that produce tension, particularly in the back, the neck, and the spine. Practitioners help individuals become aware of unhealthy postures by observing how they walk, sit, and move during everyday movements; they then provide instruction for more efficient movement that reduces tension and pain. Preliminary evaluation shows that this technique can help improve chronic back pain more effectively than home-based general exercise.[5]

Spinal Manipulation

Chiropractors use quick, sharp movements to align the spine. Some data show that *chiropractic manipulation* may temporarily alleviate migraine and other headaches; other studies produced mixed results regarding its efficiency for back and neck pain. Chiropractors are not medical doctors and are not licensed to prescribe medications. *Osteopathic manipulation* is similar, though more gentle than chiropractic manipulation. These practitioners focus on coaxing, rather than pushing muscles and joints beyond the spine to improve range of motion and relieve stiffness and pain. Doctors of Osteopathic Medicine are physicians who are licensed to provide treatment, prescribe drugs, and perform surgery.

Less Weight, Less Pain

Physical pain and emotional stress. Immobility and inactivity. Poor diet. Added together, these factors contribute to excess weight and are a recipe for a health disaster. By now, we should all be aware of the dangers of obesity. It wreaks widespread bodily damage and raises the likelihood of numerous health issues. Packing on extra pounds stresses the cardiovascular system and is hard on the ankles, knees, and hips. If you have arthritis in those joints, extra weight can make movement more difficult and more painful.

Almost 70 percent of Americans are either overweight or obese.[6] The links between obesity and pain are many. Excess fat triggers physiological processes that promote inflammation and pain, and people who carry more weight are physically less active. They are also more likely to be depressed. Having a higher *body mass index* (BMI)—the ratio of a person's height to weight—is an indicator for more health problems, including pain and increased risk for early mortality.[7] A higher BMI also brings a greater likelihood of more severe symptoms and a decreased quality of life among people with degenerative disc disease and fibromyalgia, as it does with other painful conditions.[8]

A Gallup Organization poll of more than 1 million Americans is the largest examination of the relationship between obesity and pain, and it shows that pain levels increase proportionately with weight gain. According to BMI scoring, 38 percent of respondents were overweight and 25 percent were obese. The overweight group reported 20 percent higher rates of pain compared to those of normal weight; obese individuals had pain that was 68 to 254 percent greater, depending on their BMI. The link between obesity and pain was stronger for women and older Americans.[9] (The relationship between obesity and pain persisted even after researchers accounted for the influences of other pain-causing health problems.)

The Magic Formula for Losing Weight

Countless diets are marketed as surefire ways to attain the ideal weight. If you need to shed weight, trendy get-skinny-quick diets are a waste of your time; when the diet ends, the weight is likely to return. The difficult part is to maintain your desired weight in the long term. Your best bet for healthy, sustainable weight loss is to make lifestyle changes that increase activity and reduce calories. Eat moderate portions of satisfying, nutritious foods and get plenty of exercise on most days. The National Weight Control Registry (www.nwcr.ws), an organization that investigates characteristics of people who have successfully maintained long-term weight loss, identified common long-term strategies of individuals who lost 30 pounds or more without regaining it within a year (45 percent of the registry participants lost weight on their own; the rest dropped pounds with a weight-loss program). These are characteristics of the successful individuals:

- They eat breakfast every day.
- They exercise an average of one hour daily.
- They watch less than 10 hours of television per week.
- They weigh themselves at least once weekly.
- They are conscious of their calorie intake (they do not eat more on weekends or during vacations).

The Nutrition Connection

Poor diet is a major contributor to the leading causes of chronic disease and death in the United States, including heart disease, diabetes, and stroke.[10] Good nutrition is necessary for overall health, but despite marketing hype and Internet myth, no particular food or diet will cure a chronic disorder or completely resolve pain. What you eat can indirectly affect pain, and in some cases, food triggers make certain painful conditions worse. Eating the right kinds of foods in appropriate portions is advantageous for anyone; it is especially important to help a body in pain counteract stress and fatigue and replace nutrients that are depleted by medication. It is not always easy to make healthy eating choices, particularly when frustration or depression prompt emotional eating or when pain suppresses your motivation to make smart choices in the grocery store. A diet of lean protein, legumes, whole grains, and a variety of fruits and vegetables of different colors supplies the nutrients our bodies need to fuel energy and lower the risk for disease.

It is wise to eat packaged and processed foods only in moderation or avoid them altogether. These foods typically contain high levels of salt, sugar, chemicals, and additives that may detrimentally affect chronic conditions. Several studies have linked preservatives and some sweeteners to chronic pain. Most packaged and baked goods contain one if not the other, reinforcing the concept that eating mostly plant-based fresh foods is not only good for overall health but may be better for pain as well.

Alcohol is a depressant and a poor combination with pain. It slows central nervous system activity, disrupts sleep, and interacts dangerously with many prescription and over-the-counter medications. Drinking more than minimal amounts of any alcoholic beverage can be problematic. For some people, any amount may be too much. Long-term excessive drinking can damage the nerves and cause alcoholic neuropathy.

Fats are not all equal. Our bodies need omega-3 and omega-6 essential fatty acids but cannot produce them on their own. Western diets typically supply these fats in the wrong proportion: we eat too many omega-6 fats, which increase biological signs of inflammation, and too few omega-3 fats, which have numerous heart and brain benefits. Omega-3 fatty acids are found in sardines, trout, salmon, and other cold-water fish, as well as in flaxseeds, chia seeds, soybeans, and walnuts. Polyunsaturated oils made from corn, safflower, and sunflowers (staple ingredients in many packaged foods) are sources of omega-6 fats.

Most research on omega-3 fats and pain have involved people with rheumatoid arthritis. Studies by researchers in Scotland and England indicate that increased levels of omega-3 fats reduce related pain and swelling. Patients who took NSAIDs for rheumatoid arthritis pain were separated into groups that also took either cod liver oil capsules or a placebo for 12 weeks. At that point, they were asked to cut back or eliminate their use of NSAIDs but continue taking the cod liver oil (or the placebo). After nine months, 39 percent of participants in the cod liver oil group were able to decrease their use of NSAIDs, compared to just 10 percent of the placebo group.[11] Other studies have produced similar conclusions, some showing that patients who took fish oil reduced or discontinued their use of NSAIDs and disease-modifying anti-rheumatic drugs without painful consequences.[12] The anti-inflammatory effect of omega-3 fats might strengthen osteoarthritis-weakened cartilage, but few large-scale studies have looked closely at this potential. In a British study, guinea pigs that were prone to osteoarthritis developed healthier cartilage and improved symptoms after eating an omega-3-rich diet. A 2006 survey found that daily fish oil supplements decreased pain symptoms in 60 percent of arthritis patients.[13]

Omega-3 levels can be increased through diet. The American Heart Association recommends eating a 3.5-ounce serving of omega-3-rich fatty fish at least twice weekly. Getting enough to make a difference in your arthritis will probably require supplementation. Your doctor can determine whether fish oil supplements are advisable. If you take them, read product labels carefully to ensure that the capsules you buy contain sufficient amounts of docosahexaenoic acid (DHA) and eicosapentaenoic acid per dose. (When taking any kind of supplement, look for reputable brands.) The FDA does not regulate the sale of dietary supplements, so labels may not accurately reflect information about side effects, proper dosage, and the amount of an active ingredient. Manmade *trans fats,* or partially hydrogenated oils, are often added to stick margarine, snack foods, and packaged food products to prolong shelf life. (Even though most trans fats have been removed from many prepared foods, some products still contain them.) These are liquid vegetable oils that are solidified by processing with hydrogen. Trans fats are dangerous because they raise levels of bad cholesterol and lower good cholesterol. They also increase the risk of heart disease, stroke, and type 2 diabetes. Some evidence also links consumption of these fats with increased physiological indicators of inflammation.[14]

Dietary Recommendations for Chronic Pain Conditions

Analyzing the long-term effects of diet is difficult, and with few exceptions, little conclusive evidence links specific foods or diets to chronic diseases. Some connections, however, have been identified. In other cases, evidence is building toward potential links between food and pain.

- The National Fibromyalgia Research Association recommends limiting or eliminating red meat, refined sugar, caffeine, alcohol, fried foods, and highly processed foods. People who have fibromyalgia and other individuals with a hypersensitivity to pain may also suffer because of the intake of aspartame, a common artificial sweetener in sodas, candies, and other sugar-free food. Aspartame is an *excitotoxin;* it overactivates neurons that can heighten pain sensitivity. People who have fibromyalgia often feel better when they limit or eliminate their soda intake or follow a vegan diet of mostly raw foods, avoiding gluten and lactose.
- Effective gout medications limit the need for a strict diet, yet it is still important to understand how your eating and drinking habits can affect your symptoms. Overindulging in high-purine foods has long been thought to encourage gout, but not all foods in this category carry equal risk. A 12-year prospective analysis of more than 47,000 men revealed that consuming high levels of seafood and meats (especially organ meats) raises gout risk, while high consumption of low-fat dairy products decreases risk and reduces uric acid levels. Moderate intake of purine-rich vegetables did not affect risk.[15] People who have gout are often advised to avoid all alcoholic beverages, because they interfere with the body's ability to remove uric acid. The 12-year study identified a distinction there as well: the risk of developing gout increased with the type of alcohol and the amount consumed. Men who overindulged in beer, which has more purines than other types

of alcoholic beverages, had a particularly high risk for gout. Moderate wine consumption did not increase the risk.[16] Sugar also proved to be problematic. Drinking fruit juice and eating apples, oranges, and other high-fructose fruits increased the likelihood of developing gout, as did sugar-sweetened soft drinks. Diet soft drinks did not have the same effect.[17]

- Irritable bowel syndrome may be caused by a decline in healthful bacteria in the gastrointestinal system, either because of a poor diet or as a result of taking certain medications. People who have irritable bowel syndrome tend to be sensitive to dairy products; these and other foods can make them feel worse. For many people, gradually adding more dietary fiber or taking a fiber supplement, drinking more liquids, and eating smaller meals minimize their symptoms. (A higher fiber intake may not be recommended for patients with some gastrointestinal disorders or bacterial overgrowth syndrome.) Taking *probiotics,* which are live beneficial bacteria, helps to restore healthy bacteria. Probiotics are found in some yogurts and are available as supplements.

- Managing arthritis symptoms with dietary changes is an enticing idea; unfortunately, no particular dietary regimen has been shown to prevent, alleviate, or cure arthritis. None of the books and products that promise a cure by eliminating entire food groups or taking high doses of supplements are backed by substantial scientific studies. One proven correlation between food and arthritis is the inflammatory response caused by too many omega-6 fatty acids. High-sugar snacks and beverages may also promote inflammation. Arthritis experts recommend a balanced diet and weight control as the best approach.

- *Osteoporosis* causes bones to become thin and susceptible to fractures. The condition itself is not painful, but it can lead to spinal compression fractures or hip fractures that create moderate to severe pain in the back and legs. Recommended dietary steps include controlling salt intake to decrease bone loss and eating more foods that are rich in calcium, magnesium, vitamin D, and potassium to promote bone health. Weight-bearing exercise is also important to minimize bone loss and build new bone mass.

Identifying Food Triggers

Despite the lack of conclusive evidence relating diet to pain, many patients report improved symptoms when they avoid certain foods. Allergic reactions or sensitivities to certain foods can cause painful flare-ups. A food allergy prompts the immune system to create antibodies (and disagreeable symptoms) that encourage inflammation. Once your body makes antibodies against a specific food, the next time you consume that food, your body will react in the same way. If your joint pain is caused by celiac disease (an intestinal autoimmune disorder characterized by an inflammatory reaction to gluten), for example, it is important to avoid foods containing wheat, spelt, rye, and barley. (Fortunately, gluten-free products are widely available.) Food sensitivities cause reactions that do not involve antibodies—people who are sensitive to sweeteners, particularly high-fructose corn syrup and aspartame, feel better when they avoid them.

Despite what you may have heard, no single food affects all migraine sufferers, but many foods are migraine instigators for some people, including the following:

- aged cheeses, smoked products, red wine, yeast, and some beans that contain tyramine, a chemical compound
- fermented, salted, or pickled foods
- caffeine
- dairy products
- bacon, salami, ham, hot dogs, and other cured meats that contain nitrites

Monosodium glutamate (MSG), a high-sodium flavor enhancer, is added to many canned, prepackaged, and restaurant foods. Ancient Romans were avid consumers of MSG, which they made from decomposed fish and salt. Modern MSG is created differently: by adding sodium to excreted glutamic acid from genetically engineered bacteria. How MSG affects people continues to be hotly debated. Some people believe it is an addictive substance that triggers headaches, joint pain, heart palpitations, and other problems. Others consider it to be only an additive that makes food taste better. While the World Health Organization, the American Medical Association, and other prestigious panels consider MSG to be safe for the general public, many people appear to be sensitive to the substance.

Physicians at Oregon Health & Science University conducted an intriguing experiment to determine whether MSG affects pain. They put 57 patients who had fibromyalgia and irritable bowel syndrome on a four-week diet that excluded MSG and aspartame. Among the 37 people who completed the diet, 84 percent reported a decrease in painful symptoms and better quality of life. Those individuals (the ones who improved) then participated in a secondary double-blind, placebo-controlled trial. Over two weeks, they were given either MSG or a placebo for three consecutive days. Individuals in the MSG group displayed a significant return of symptoms.[18] MSG is also a component of hydrolyzed protein, yeast extract, and autolyzed yeast. If you are sensitive to MSG, read food labels carefully to avoid these ingredients, as well as glutamic acid. Whatever it is called, MSG is added to more foods than you might imagine.

Tracking Food Triggers

Maintaining a food diary can help you identify foods that trigger pain or other undesirable symptoms. Record everything you eat and drink, no matter how small the quantity. Try eliminating troublesome foods from your diet for 30 days, then gradually reintroduce them one by one to determine whether any of them make your symptoms worse.

Calcium, Vitamin D, and Magnesium

The body uses numerous vitamins and minerals to complete complex biological functions. Three of these elements, calcium, vitamin D, and magnesium, are emerging as potential powerhouses for overall health. Having a deficiency in any one of them may adversely affect pain.

Most people know that calcium is a structural component for strong bones and teeth; it is also necessary for development of soft tissue, blood vessels, and cellular fluids. Having a calcium deficiency creates brittle bones and contributes to joint pain. Vitamin D is also necessary. It helps the body absorb calcium, modulates cell growth, and works against inflammation. (The skin converts the sun's ultraviolet rays to vitamin D; exposing your skin to sunlight for just 15 minutes a day is sufficient— exposure time varies with a person's age, skin type, geographic location, and season.) While we do not completely understand all the nuances of how vitamin D affects the body, a flurry of research in the past few years points to a potential link between inadequate levels of vitamin D and various painful conditions. Individuals with fibromyalgia in small Egyptian and Saudi Arabian studies who were treated with high doses of vitamin D experienced widespread symptom improvement.[19] A much larger review that used data from the 2001-4 U.S. National Health and Nutrition Examination Survey found that 81 percent of adults with diabetes were deficient in vitamin D. Among pain patients treated with morphine at the Mayo Clinic, individuals who were lacking in vitamin D required 48 percent more morphine each day than patients with adequate levels of vitamin D.[20]

We are also finding that magnesium plays a more significant role in the body than we have previously understood. Every bodily organ needs magnesium to function properly, so it is understandable that low levels of this trace mineral may be responsible for many different symptoms. Whole grains, nuts, and green vegetables increase the levels of magnesium. Numerous dietary and health conditions decrease magnesium, including too much coffee, soda, alcohol, or salt in the diet. Diuretics and some medications may also lower absorption. Individuals who have diabetes, kidney disease, or hyperthyroidism may need magnesium supplements; people with gluten sensitivity or irritable bowel syndrome often have difficulty absorbing magnesium or lose it through diarrhea.

Magnesium may also have a starring role in pain relief by regulating nerve functions and blocking NMDA receptors that heighten pain sensitivity. Not enough convincing research supports widespread use of magnesium therapy for pain. Initial research, however, shows that it appears to lower pain from migraines, complex regional pain syndrome

(CRPS), and neuropathy (intravenous magnesium has been used to relieve nerve pain associated with pancreatic cancer).[21] Other scientific findings link magnesium deficiency to migraines, asthma, and allergies, which may explain why so many people have all three conditions. Migraine sufferers tend to have lower levels of magnesium compared to those with tension-type headaches or no headaches at all, and some studies suggest that magnesium supplements may shorten the duration of migraines or prevent them. Sufficient magnesium intake may also lessen muscle spasms and back pain.

People who have fibromyalgia often lack sufficient amounts of magnesium, and their symptoms—fatigue, stiff or cramped muscles, irritability, and sleeping problems—parallel indications of magnesium deficiency. (Theoretically, when magnesium levels drop, levels of substance P increase and nerves fire too easily, even from minor stimuli.)[22] Much of the research regarding the relationship between magnesium and pain has focused on this population. A small-scale study conducted more than 20 years ago suggested a potential benefit when fibromyalgia patients were given magnesium. A few studies, though not definitive, found that magnesium combined with malic acid, calcium, or an antidepressant blocks pain and muscle tenderness.[23] Research in this area is scarce, not sufficient to define an appropriate dosage.

More information about calcium, vitamin D, and magnesium can be found at the website of the National Institutes of Health, which provides information about dietary supplements (http://ods.od.nih.gov). Another source of information is the Office of Dietary Supplements at the NIH website, which lists recommended daily amounts and sources of vitamins, minerals, and supplements (http://ods.od.nih.gov/factsheets/list-VitaminsMinerals).

Injections, Implants, and Neurostimulators

When medications and other therapies leave patients with high levels of residual pain, secondary alternatives may provide measurable pain relief. Numbing injections are helpful for many people. Implantable devices that displace and disrupt pain messages provide longer-lasting relief for individuals with severe, treatment-resistant pain.

Injections and Nerve Blocks

Injury or centralization—the impact that pain has on the brain and spinal cord—often makes nerves more sensitive so that they signal pain with less provocation. When nerve pain cannot be relieved with oral medications or other therapies, injecting local anesthetics (with or without steroids) onto or near nerves may temporarily provide relief. Even when the initial dramatic relief wears off, many patients experience long-lasting, partial residual relief. Injections delivered directly into painful trigger points are a viable method of supplementing physical therapy for chronically tense or twitching muscles.

Prolotherapy is a rather unusual approach to pain reduction. A concentrated dextrose (sugar-water) solution is injected into or around ligaments (the joint tissue that connects bones) or tendons (the tissue that connects muscle to bones) to produce local inflammation. ("Prolo" refers to proliferation, because the treatment speeds the growth of new ligament tissue.) The injections appear to prompt the body's wound-healing response, stimulating tissue repair by increasing blood supply, collagen, and other nutrients at the site. Collagen shrinks as it matures, tightening and strengthening the area. Prolotherapy is not standard by any means, and some physicians dismiss it as quackery or a placebo. Others say their patients have good results after a few months of injections. Five studies of different types of prolotherapy concluded that it helped low-back pain only when it was combined with other treatments.[24] It is unclear what produced these positive results: a placebo effect, the injected solution, or simply the act of inserting a needle into deep tissue. Other studies found that it reduced pain no more than injections of saline (placebo) did.

While the jury may still be out on prolotherapy, we have more data and experience with *nerve blocks,* injections of medication that abate abnormal firing of sensitive nerves. Administering a block is a relatively simple process and a particularly effective method of calming hypersensitive nerves. It is the same procedure dentists use to numb a nerve before filling a tooth or performing a root canal. For chronic pain, injections of local anesthetics, steroids, or opioids into a facet joint or the space around the nerves may interrupt the pain cycle and relax the nervous system. Depending on the type of block and many other factors, relief can last several hours or permanently. Nerve blocks are particularly effective when combined with other treatment approaches. They are not always the best treatment for a pain problem; some people experience dramatic relief, but others do not.

Blocking specific nerves reduces sensitivity to pain, especially if the underlying source of irritation can be resolved. The *sympathetic nervous system* runs in chains along the spine and branches out in fine nets of nerves toward different parts of the body, where it regulates blood flow, sweating, and glandular function. These nerves appear to play an important role in neuropathic pain, especially complex regional pain syndrome (CRPS) (see chapter 2). Nerve-block injections at the portion of the sympathetic chain in the neck are often part of the treatment of CRPS affecting the arm or hand, and injections at the portion of the sympathetic chain in the low back are often used to treat CRPS of the leg or foot (figure 5.1). The *peripheral nervous system* enables the body's voluntary and involuntary nervous functions (table 5.1). These nerves cause chronic pain when they become irritated or injured.

Headaches that spread from the back of the neck toward the forehead

TABLE 5.1   Examples of common nerve blocks

Location of pain	Affected nerves
Sympathetic nerves	
Legs or feet	Lumbar sympathetic (front of spine in lower back) (figure 5.1)
Face, arms, or hands	Stellate ganglion (front of the spine in lower neck) (figure 5.1)
Abdomen	Celiac plexus (abdomen)
Pelvis	Superior hypogastric plexus (in front of the S1 portion of the sacrum) and ganglion impar (in front of the coccyx)
Peripheral nerves	
Head	Occipital (base of the neck to the back of the head)
Chest	Intercostal
Pelvis	Ilioinguinal (front of the lower abdomen)

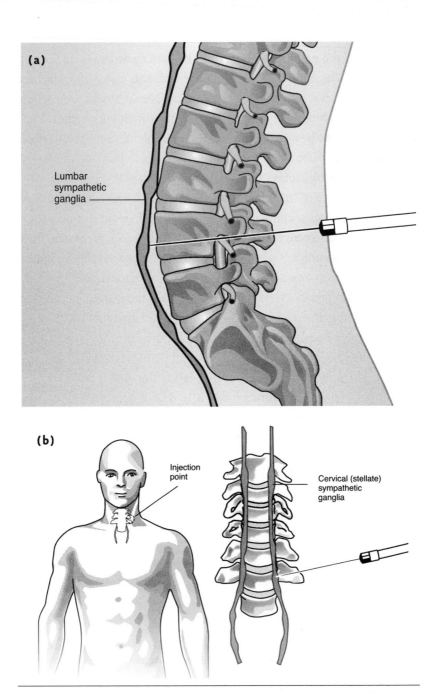

FIGURE 5.1. Nerve blocks are administered to the lumbar sympathetic ganglia to reduce neuropathic pain of the leg or foot (*above*), and to the cervical (stellate) sympathetic ganglia to reduce neuropathic pain in the arm or hand (*below*).

may occur when peripheral *occipital nerves* are irritated by neck injuries, muscle spasm, or arthritic changes in the cervical spine. Occipital nerve blocks with steroids often successfully treat this type of headache. Blocking, burning, or freezing the *intercostal nerves* can lessen neural pain in the chest wall, including postmastectomy pain. Blocks are also used to calm the *ilioinguinal nerve,* which affects part of the groin and pubic area; it can become damaged during surgery or by scar tissue that develops after a hernia repair or a cesarean section.

For the past three years, nerve blocks have been both friend and foe in my fight against complex regional pain syndrome. In theory, each block is meant to build upon the previous one, overlapping to give longer relief. My experience has been a bit of a roller-coaster ride, since I seem to reach a plateau with both blocks. Bier nerve blocks that first squeeze the blood from my lower leg and then administer a combination of drugs into a vein in my foot have worked the best, giving me about three weeks without pain, but the mechanics of this type of block are a problem. Putting a large needle into my foot, which is already compromised by CRPS, is less than ideal, and eventually the blocks begin hurting, not helping. Lumbar sympathetic blocks are far less stressful for me; they are also less effective. At times, these have also given me close to three weeks of relief. I've had other problems, like an infected ingrown toenail, which might have limited the effects of the block, or the block just stopped working. Currently, I have one block or the other every couple of weeks. If the Bier block doesn't work or my foot gives me a sign that it's time to switch, I have the lumbar sympathetic block. I have a pretty good quality of life between blocks. I'm able to get around more freely and enjoy little things like taking a walk or going to the movies. These pain-free weeks are a gift that I hope will grow. For now I just feel blessed to have them.

—Suzi

....

The most common nerve block is the *epidural steroid injection* (figure 5.2), which delivers a steroid and sometimes a local anesthetic to subdue inflammation around irritated nerves. Epidural injections are administered to the lumbar portion of the spine to relieve radiating leg pain from sciatica or other conditions and to the cervical spine when symptoms extend into the arms. They are particularly effective for nerve-root irritation caused by a herniated disc but are less successful for the diagnoses of spinal stenosis and widespread degeneration of the spine. Thoracic (in the chest) epidural steroid injections calm pain associated with thoracic shingles, decreasing the risk of postherpetic neuralgia. If you have sciatica on either the left or the right side (but not both), a *transforaminal epidural steroid injection,* given at the side of the spine where the affected nerve root is, may be more beneficial than a traditional epidural injection, which is typically administered in the middle of the back—this is still a controversial issue. The effects of steroid injections last several

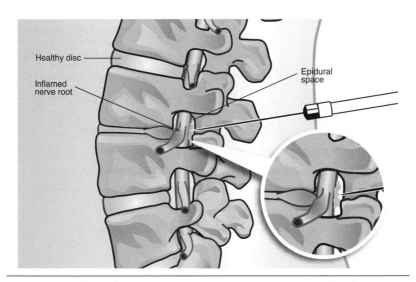

FIGURE 5.2. Epidural steroid injections deliver a corticosteroid and a local anesthetic into the epidural space to reduce inflammation around irritated nerves.

weeks or much longer, depending on the underlying problem. We limit them to just a few per year because overuse can weaken the spine and surrounding tissues and suppresses the body's natural hormonal balance.

> ### CRITERIA FOR AN
> ### IMPLANTABLE PAIN DEVICE
>
> When more conservative therapies have failed, a pain pump may be considered for patients who have no substance abuse problem, no chronic or active infection, no uncontrolled bleeding disorder, and no psychological or medical issues that preclude having a pump.

Implantable Pain Pumps

Oral analgesics are a blessing for many of us, but they have a drawback: they diffuse throughout the body before they reach the spinal cord, where they are needed most. An *intrathecal pain pump* solves the problem by delivering a single drug or a combination of drugs directly into the cerebrospinal fluid, which flows around the spine and the brain. In a procedure that usually takes about three hours, a pump the size of a small bagel is surgically implanted under the abdominal skin, connected to a catheter that goes into the spine and the spinal fluid, and is programmed to slowly release medication. (The unit can also be programmed to release adjusted doses during the day.) Because it delivers medicine precisely to the spinal cord, the pump causes fewer side effects and provides better pain relief than oral analgesics. A pain pump also requires less medication: morphine delivered in this way is 300 times as strong as it would be if taken orally. Pumps usually need to be filled every one to three months by inserting a syringe through the skin and into the pump. A psychological assessment can help to determine a person's emotional readiness for such technology. A trial treatment phase is often implemented to determine whether the pump effectively decreases pain without significant side effects. If that works, a permanent implant can be installed. Although it is not the answer for everyone, a pain pump can effectively resolve pain with few side effects for some people.

SPINAL PUMP

MARY, AGE 52, EXPERIENCED INTENSE PAIN in her right shoulder and arm following a mastectomy and a radiation treatment two years earlier. The treatment appeared to have successfully contained her breast cancer, but Mary's postoperative pain worsened, and she continued to lose strength and mobility in her arm. We suspected that Mary's pain was related to tumor involvement of the brachial plexus nerves, which emerge from the neck and provide all motor and sensory function to the arm, a diagnosis that was confirmed by a PET scan. Mary then began a new course of chemotherapy to treat the residual tumor, but her pain intensified and her arm remained weak.

We began treating Mary's pain with a combination of anti-inflammatories, neuropathic drugs, and opioids. We also tried antiseizure and antidepressant medications. This regimen was somewhat helpful, but significant pain remained. The next step was a series of injections into the brachial plexus nerves, which successfully blocked the neuropathic pain signals for several weeks. After the third injection, it was apparent that this method would not provide lasting relief, so a more aggressive measure was necessary: implanting an electric stimulator into the spine. After careful consideration, Mary agreed this was her best hope for long-term pain relief. We fitted her with a trial stimulator, first inserting needles into the spine of her neck where the brachial plexus nerves branch away from the spinal cord. Wires were then threaded through the needle; the other end of the wires exited the skin and connected to a temporary stimulator pack that Mary carried with her. The stimulation worked well, reducing Mary's pain by about half, but the remaining pain was still severe, so she decided to supplement the stimulator with a spinal pain pump. When Mary returned to the hospital, we inserted a catheter into her spine and administered a trial combination of Dilaudid, Clonidine, and Bupivacaine. After two days, Mary was very pleased with the result. So, during another minor surgery, we installed the pump under her abdominal skin, with a catheter positioned into the spinal fluid to facilitate direct infusion of medicine. We made a few postsurgical adjustments to increase the dose. One month later, with the combination of the pump and the stimulator, Mary reported a 90 percent reduction of pain. After a year, she continued to have very low pain levels. ☺

Noninvasive and Invasive Neurostimulation

Neurostimulators perform like pacemakers for pain. A person self-regulates the delivery of a mild electrical current into the spine as needed. The current acts as a kind of white noise against pain. Some people who use them feel a tingling sensation instead of pain; others say their pain is simply less noticeable.

A noninvasive *transcutaneous electrical nerve stimulation* (TENS) unit scrambles pain messages in the spinal cord. A TENS unit transmits low-voltage electrical impulses through the skin, stimulating nerves and replacing painful sensations with a mild tingling. The unit consists of a battery-powered device with flat electrode pads that adhere to the skin above the point of pain. The person with chronic pain uses a small remote-control unit to switch the device on and off and to control the strength and length of the impulses. A review of studies involving more than 1,200 individuals confirmed the effectiveness of TENS for chronic musculoskeletal pain.[25] American Academy of Neurology guidelines advise that TENS can help diabetic neuropathy, although it fails to benefit patients with chronic low-back pain. TENS can provide hours of relief, depending on the nature and severity of the pain. Because tolerance may develop with constant use, the unit should not be used for more than a few hours per day. Many people find that it continues to reduce pain for some time after it is turned off. Other types of neurostimulators, including microcurrent electrical neuromuscular stimulators (MENS), H-wave stimulators, and interferential stimulators work in a similar way.

More powerful neurostimulators can be implanted into the spine or under the skin. Spinal-cord stimulators are used more frequently than pain pumps for severe pain because they are effective without many of the risks: they do not become blocked or need to be refilled, and there is less potential for infection. The stimulation unit is connected to thin, spaghetti-like wires that are threaded up through the epidural space to overlay the portion of the spinal cord where pain signals originate (figure 5.3).

An implanted spinal or peripheral stimulator may be the next step for patients who continue to have back, leg, or arm pain after spinal surgery (or when surgery is not recommended). Patients with CRPS or localized

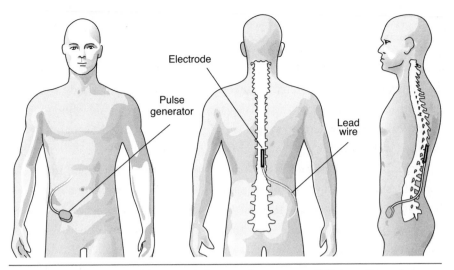

FIGURE 5.3. Electrical stimulation travels from a pulse generator (*left*) to an electrode (*center*) through fine wires that are positioned in the epidural space above the area of pain.

neuralgias also respond well to this treatment. Success rates with peripheral neuropathies or phantom-limb pain are lower, but a trial with a stimulator is still worthwhile if the pain has not responded to other treatments. Unlike other invasive treatments, a temporary stimulator can be tested before a permanent device is installed. A trial electrode is inserted and connected to an external power supply that is left in place for about a week. If the temporary electrode curtails pain sufficiently, it is replaced with a permanent electrode that is charged by an internal battery under the skin. If not, the device and the electrodes are removed.

Peripheral-nerve stimulation produces weak electrical impulses that close the pain gate. The electrode wire is inserted under the skin of the painful area, rather than into the spine. Many patients can then reduce or eliminate their pain medication. Abdominal pain, postherpetic neuralgia, and other neuropathic pain conditions can be treated successfully this way. Peripheral-nerve stimulation is quite safe and is usually performed as an outpatient procedure under a local anesthetic. Complications are rare but may include infection or pain at the incision or at the location of the electrodes or the power pack. Although it is not a common occurrence, nearby blood vessels or nerves can be accidentally damaged by the wire. Some patients say that the shifting of the electrodes or the power pack is a bit uncomfortable.

. . . .

My facial pain from trigeminal neuralgia began after surgery on my left eye. Instead of decreasing, the post-op pain increased and radiated throughout the entire left side of my face, lower jaw, and above my eyebrow. It was a constant burning; I've never known such pain in my life. I'm an avid reader, and when the neuralgia began, I could not comprehend what I was reading. I felt as though I was going out of my mind, and for a while I was afraid that I was developing Alzheimer's. Everything revolved around my pain. My husband and I no longer had a social life or any type of intimacy, which was very hard on both of us. Different medications were unsuccessful and gave me no relief. Acupuncture worked for a few hours but did not last. One doctor tried a nerve block, which only intensified the pain. Then I saw the doctors at the University of Southern California. First they tried Gamma Knife surgery, a type of minimally invasive precise radiation therapy used to treat tumors and other abnormalities in the brain. That helped somewhat, but I still had a lot of pain, but I never gave up hope. Then I had a new procedure, a facial stimulator that has helped so much. I still have ongoing pain, but it is at a level I can handle. The downside is having to turn the stimulator off at night so that my body does not become accustomed to it. I wake up in the morning with increased pain and have to wait for my medication and the stimulator to take effect, but it has given me my life back.
—Julie
. . . .

Occipital nerve stimulation works in the same way. A thin wire inserted beneath the skin at the base of the skull is connected to a power source implanted under the collarbone or in the abdomen that sends electrical impulses to the occipital nerve. The wire may also be placed to combat other types of pain: under the skin of the forehead for headaches that tend to occur in the front of the head, or under the skin of the cheek and jaw for patients with trigeminal neuralgia or facial pain. At the onset of pain, patients activate a small remote control to release a minimal electrical current that disrupts pain signals. The procedure works well for some patients, but we still lack data from well-controlled long-term studies of occipital nerve stimulation, even though the procedure has been available for several years. A few small studies suggest that the procedure slows the intensity and frequency of migraine and cluster headaches that do not respond to medication. How the stimulation reduces pain is not well defined; it may restore balance in a hypersensitive central pain system.

. . . .

At 83 years old, I was blessed with generally good health and an active life. That all changed when I developed terrible headaches out of the blue. Throughout my life I have had headaches now and then, but I had no history of serious headaches, and certainly not like this. The pain in my neck, temples, and all over my head was intense. It occurred all day, every day, and sometimes upset my stomach. For almost two years, I went from doctor to doctor, trying to find the cause of this horrible pain, and trying to relieve it. During that time, I tried many pain medications and even steroid injections in my neck. Nothing worked or even reduced the pain. Unable to do much, I spent most of my time in bed. My primary doctor referred me to a neurologist who believed that because my pain subsided when I lay down, it might be caused by a leak of my spinal fluid. He twice tried a blood patch, taking blood from my arm and injecting it into my spine to fill the leak; that didn't work.

Finally, I was referred to Dr. Richeimer, who suggested an occipital nerve stimulator. I was willing to try anything. It worked right away, as though he had turned off the pain switch. For the first time in months I was absolutely free of headache pain. The following week he swapped the temporary unit for a more permanent stimulator under the skin of my waist. Now when I feel a headache developing, I turn the unit on. I first feel the impulses going up my neck, then a tingling that lasts for 10 or 15 minutes before it stops and my pain is gone. I may need to leave the stimulator on for most of the day for stubborn pain. I've gone from terrible daily headaches that kept me bedridden to pain that I can turn off when I need to, and I take no pain medication. It's a miracle that has given my life back to me.

—Ida

. . . .

One of the most effective methods of treating epilepsy and Parkinson's disease also holds promise for some chronic pain syndromes. *Deep brain stimulation* (DBS) may provide long-term relief from complex regional pain syndrome, pain in the lower back and legs, and neuropathic peripheral pain that does not respond to other therapies. People who have phantom-limb pain also respond well to this therapy.[26] It has been less effective for people who have spinal cord injuries, pain after stroke, or other painful syndromes involving the central nervous system. DBS alleviates pain by delivering electrical pulses to areas of the brain that process pain signals. Electrodes are implanted into specific areas of the brain (this requires drilling small holes in the skull) and a small electric generator is placed under the skin of the chest or the abdomen.

Ongoing research is exploring *repetitive transcranial magnetic stimulation* (rTMS), a noninvasive method that uses an electromagnet coil on the scalp to reduce pain. The device generates low-frequency magnetic pulses to stimulate a specific small area of mood-regulating nerve cells in the brain. rTMS is FDA-approved to treat major depression in patients who do not respond to medication, and it is of great interest to the pain community. If it works well, it will be the first method to manipulate brain neurons without using electrodes (or medications). Initial research shows that a single rTMS session can produce short-term relief for myofascial pain syndrome and that repeated sessions over several days may hold promise for short- and moderate-term relief of other types of neuropathic pain.[27]

Destroying Nerves and Tissue for Relief

When treating neuropathic pain, we try as much as possible to avoid destroying nerves. However, sometimes it is necessary to do just that when intolerable pain resists all other treatments. We destroy the troublesome nerve with chemical injections of phenol or pure ethanol, or we use needles that kill nerves with cold or heat. *Radiofrequency ablation* is an option for relieving some types of neck and back pain when medication and physical therapy fail. The first step is a fluoroscopically guided diagnostic injection of numbing medicine to identify whether the small spinal facet joints are the source of pain. Then a small fluoroscopy-guided probe applies radiofrequency energy to the nerve or nerves that carry the pain signals from the offending joint or joints. The energy will kill or stun these small nerves. Radiofrequency nerve ablation is minimally invasive and is usually performed as an outpatient procedure under local anesthesia (or with mild sedation). Nerves eventually regenerate, so unless the underlying condition improves, pain usually returns over the next 9–12 months as the nerves grow back.

For most patients, radiofrequency ablation carries less risk and is preferable to injections of a nerve-killing chemical that may further irritate the nerve or spread beyond the source of pain. *Pulsed radiofrequency* administers the same kind of energy in brief bursts to treat peripheral-nerve pain. The tissue does not heat up as much as it does with radiofrequency—the nerve is stunned rather than killed. Compared to radiofrequency ablation, the positive effects of pulsed radiofrequency do not last as long. The nerves recuperate in just three to six months, compared to approximately a year after radiofrequency ablation, but the safety profile is better.

Intradiscal Procedures

Traditionally, degenerative disc diseases that do not respond to medication, rest, or epidural injections have been treated with highly invasive surgery to decompress pressure on spinal nerves. Sometimes these procedures can cause more pain and disability than the patient suffered before the surgery, so the decision for surgical intervention should always be approached cautiously. Fortunately, newer, minimally invasive outpatient procedures performed under mild sedation reduce the risk and the recovery time associated with surgery. These nonsurgical decompression procedures remove or dissolve disc material to relieve pressure on spinal nerves; they treat the cause of spinal disc problems, rather than the symptoms. Decompression treatment offers an alternative when other, nonsurgical treatments fail to alleviate pain. These procedures have a low complication rate; however, the long-term rate of success is not yet clear.

Replacing Open Surgery with Less Invasive Procedures

Open disectomy is performed under general anesthesia to remove herniated disc material that presses on the spinal cord or a nerve root. Working through a long incision in the back, the surgeon cuts the muscles away from the bone and removes a portion (or all) of the herniated disc material. Thankfully, newer microsurgeries accomplish the same goal without jeopardizing nerve roots or the spinal cord. During a *microdiscectomy,* muscles are moved out of the way rather than cut. The procedure is performed through a one-inch incision and recovery is quicker and less painful; patients go home the same day or stay one night in the hospital. Some people develop a new herniation in the same disc after microdiscectomy; disc fusion or replacement with artificial disc material may be recommended for patients who have recurrences. *Lumbar endoscopic discectomy* is performed under intravenous sedation and local anesthesia. Using x-ray guidance and a video endoscope, microsurgical tools are inserted into the disc through a small incision. In a matter of minutes, the damaged disc material is cut out or pulverized with a high-powered jet of saline solution and then suctioned away; the remainder of the disc is left intact. *Nucleoplasty* and *discoplasty* use laser or radiofrequency energy to destroy some of the disc material and reduce the disc protrusion. Pain relief usually occurs within days after the procedure.

Percutaneous discectomy (also called *percutaneous disc decompression*) works particularly well for mildly compressed, unruptured discs that send radiating pain into the legs. A needlelike tube inserted through a small incision punctures the disc. Some of the disc material is removed, reducing the herniation so that it no longer rests on the nerve root. The process takes just 30 to 45 minutes and recovery is usually quick: free from the effects of general anesthesia and more invasive surgery, most patients return to work in 7 to 10 days. Subsequent physical therapy may be required to strengthen the muscles in the back and the leg.

When all other treatments fail to relieve pain from spinal stenosis, surgical intervention is the only remaining alternative. This is particularly the case with patients who have incontinence or difficulty standing or walking because of muscle weakness. Historically, such surgery has involved *laminectomy,* a highly invasive procedure to remove the lamina, the portion of the vertebra covering the spinal canal. Sometimes a spinal fusion that immobilizes two or more vertebrae is performed at the same time. Most surgeons now prefer *endoscopic laminotomy,* a less invasive procedure that accomplishes the same goal but does not require general anesthesia, a large incision, an extended hospital stay, or a long recovery. Using a fluoroscope for guidance, the surgeon inserts a fine needle into one side of the spine. When the needle is in place, the surgeon makes a one-half- to one-inch incision around the needle. The tissue and muscles over the spine are gently pulled away and a hollow surgical cylinder is secured in the space, or "channel." A tiny surgical camera is then positioned in the channel to provide an enlarged view of the problem area, and the portion of bone that is compressing the nerve is removed.

SUMMARY POINTS

- No specific diet or food is known to cure chronic pain, although individual sensitivities to certain foods may trigger pain.
- Obesity contributes to poor overall health and may intensify some painful conditions.
- Most painful conditions benefit from the right kind of active physical therapy and exercise.
- Injections, implants, and neurostimulators often help when more conservative treatment fails.

6

Complementary and Alternative Therapies

Complementary and alternative medicine (CAM) includes health systems, practices, and products that are intended to improve some aspect of health but that are not part of conventional Western medicine. *Complementary medicine* is used with conventional treatment; *alternative medicine* is used in place of it. Most CAM therapies are not well studied and many are of questionable benefit, but being termed complementary or alternative does not necessarily mean a treatment is without value, just that it falls beyond the bounds of traditional Western approaches to health and healing.

Numerous CAM treatments have their origins in ancient Indian and Asian healing arts and have been used by different cultures for thousands of years before gaining popularity in the United States. More than two-thirds of the world's population, in fact, use at least one form of complementary or alternative medicine. According to the 2007 National Health Interview Survey, 38 percent of American adults also use some type of CAM, spending nearly $34 billion on CAM products and practitioners annually. The usage figure is surely much higher now, as consumers increasingly search for ways to manage their symptoms and enhance their overall well-being (table 6.1).

Despite exaggerated and sometimes outrageous claims by manufacturers and marketers, we do not yet have evidence that any CAM therapy or product can cure disease. Nor does any single treatment work for

TABLE 6.1 Complementary and alternative medicine (CAM) in the United States

People who use CAM:	38% of adults, 12% of children
Conditions that most often prompt use:	Pain in the back, neck, and joints
Most popular CAM options:	"Natural" products (including herbal supplements, excluding vitamin and mineral supplements)
5 most popular natural products:	Fish oil supplements, glucosamine, echinacea, flaxseed oil/pills, and ginseng
Greatest 5-year increase in use:	Deep breathing, meditation, massage, and yoga

Source: National Center for Complementary and Alternative Medicine.

everyone. Nevertheless, some do aid in the reduction of stress, anxiety, and tension, which so often accompany tenacious pain. Many patients report that supplementing their pain-management strategy with one or more CAM procedures helps them to relax, refocus, and find relief.

More people use CAM for pain than for any other health concern. Millions say they find relief and comfort from at least one CAM option, yet we are not always able to explain how or why that happens. Some complementary and alternative treatments appear to relieve pain indirectly by reducing inflammation or decreasing anxiety, but little scientific evidence conclusively supports the effectiveness of most CAM therapies. Research projects are often small or poorly designed or represent case reports more than sound scientific examination. Often no control groups are used, so it is impossible to make comparative judgments about a particular therapy. Large, well-controlled studies are expensive, and funding from objective sources is limited and is more likely to be appropriated for research on conventional treatments. The National Center for Complementary and Alternative Medicine (NCCAM), a member organization of the National Institutes of Health, sponsors CAM research and provides results of clinical trials and other studies of CAM therapies (http://nccam.nih.gov and www.clinicaltrials.gov).

Safety is always an issue with any type of treatment, and it is especially important with CAM therapies because most are unregulated. Practitioners do not always need a license or certification to provide products or services. Some CAM can do harm: a yoga pose stretched too far can cause injury and pain, and some herbs and supplements may conflict with medications in unpleasant or dangerous ways. A few CAM therapies are backed by well-documented studies and are now recognized as safe and reasonable additions or alternatives to other forms of treatment, and numerous hospitals and medical centers now offer CAM programs.

Few CAM therapies have been rigorously studied. A double-blind, placebo-controlled study is the most reliable form of research. In this type of project, a group of participants uses the treatment under study, while others receive a placebo. Neither researchers nor participants know which group is using the real therapy—hence, they are both "blind" in the experiment. Thus subjectivity and the power of suggestion are eliminated from everyone involved in the trial. Size is also important—larger studies produce more reliable findings. Until a treatment is tested this way, its usefulness and safety remain inconclusive.

Energy-Based Therapies

Many CAM therapies are based on the premise that maintaining a balanced flow of the body's vital energy promotes health and well-being. Ancient healing arts refer to this essential life force by different names. It is "qi" (pronounced "chee") in traditional Chinese medicine, "prana" in Hinduism, and "mana" in the Hawaiian culture. Cultural beliefs dictate that this life energy flows to bodily organs along pathways called meridians. A constant flow of qi promotes a healthy body and mind. Stress, poor diet, and other factors block or disrupt the flow of qi, promoting illness and poor health.

Acupuncture

An *acupuncture* treatment penetrates the skin along meridians with sterilized, hair-thin needles to stimulate and rebalance qi. (The FDA regulates acupuncture needles as medical devices, as it does syringes and surgical scalpels.) Some acupuncturists apply a mild electrical current through the needles. Others use *moxibustion,* igniting dried moxa (the spongy herb known as mugwort) that is wrapped around the needle tip to generate heat and further stimulate the body's self-healing mechanisms.

Depending on the person's condition, some people experience immediate relief after one or two acupuncture sessions, but several treatments are usually necessary.

Western medicine does not recognize the existence of qi or meridians. It offers a more conventional explanation: that acupuncture improves the blood flow to tissues or stimulates the secretion of endorphins and other pain-modulating neurochemicals by the central nervous system. Some researchers suspect that meridians represent myofascial chains that connect adjacent nerves and tissues and that acupuncture sends pain-reducing signals along the fascial sheath that surrounds muscles. That would help to explain why stimulating an acupuncture point in the leg or the back affects a different area of the body. Mayo Clinic researchers supported this hypothesis with their discovery that meridians identified by Chinese documents more than 2,000 years ago coincide anatomically with areas of myofascial trigger points, indicating that acupuncture may provide a unique approach for treating chronic myofascial pain.[1] It may also work against painful arthritis. A study at the University of Arizona followed 168 patients with *temporomandibular* disorders (jaw pain caused by osteoarthritis, rheumatoid arthritis, or problems in the surrounding muscles or joint). Over an eight-week period, participants who were treated with traditional Chinese medicine (acupuncture and herbs) experienced better short-term pain relief, less interference with social activities, and improved quality of life compared to those who received

CHINESE AND JAPANESE ACUPUNCTURE

Although Chinese and Japanese acupuncture techniques share a common theoretical foundation, they are somewhat different. Chinese acupuncture, which is more common in the United States, places needles deeper and is often combined with acupressure. The Japanese method dictates the use of minimal acupuncture to prompt the body's healing process and uses smaller, thinner needles to access the body's qi (energy) just below the surface of the skin. Practitioners of Japanese acupuncture rely on touch rather than sight, using their hands to find acupressure points before the needles are inserted. Most of them also routinely use moxibustion to generate heat under the skin.

only a community-based psychosocial self-care program.[2] Regardless of the differences between Eastern and Western medical philosophies, acupuncture is widely accepted and practiced in the United States; even the U.S. Army uses it to reduce pain from combat injuries.

Numerous research projects that attempted to assess the viability of acupuncture for different types of chronic pain have produced conflicting results.

- Evidence is more conclusive for the use of acupuncture to relieve neck pain and osteoarthritis of the knee than for other conditions.
- Acupuncture procedures offer more short-term pain relief than NSAIDs for people with cervical disc pain, and its benefit is similar to that of NSAIDs in the long term.[3]
- Trials involving patients with disc herniation found that acupuncture alone relieved pain and was even more effective when combined with a nerve block. It worked as well but no better than NSAIDs among 80 study participants with radicular pain (sciatica-like pain that comes from the spinal nerve roots).[4]
- In preliminary studies, 76 percent of patients with peripheral neuropathy experienced diminished pain after acupuncture sessions, compared to 15 percent of individuals in the control group.[5] A small project at Harvard Medical School found that

Japanese-style acupuncture relieved painful diabetic neuropathy more effectively than its Chinese counterpart, while both relieved pain and improved nerve sensation.[6]

- Some findings show that acupuncture decreases symptoms of migraine, tension headaches, myofascial pain, and low-back pain as effectively as medication. Other large studies have concluded that it does not.

- Most randomized controlled trials involving the use of acupuncture for fibromyalgia did not find a benefit.

Closer analysis shows that much of the research has been of poor quality, limited size, or questionable design, making it difficult to conclude with certainty whether acupuncture can actually treat painful conditions. Although more Western physicians now recommend acupuncture to relieve pain, it remains controversial. It appears to be more effective than no treatment at all, yet a good deal of evidence hints that any realized benefit is largely a result of a placebo effect; in some cases, sham procedures that simulate acupuncture without puncturing the skin have been just as effective.[7] Millions of people who have acupuncture each year might disagree with that conclusion.

Acupressure

Traditional Chinese *acupressure* and *Shiatsu,* its Japanese counterpart, stimulate acupuncture points with gentle pressure from the fingers, knuckles, palms, or feet rather than with needles. An assessment of 9 Shiatsu studies and 71 studies of Chinese acupressure published between 1990 and 2011 concluded that despite flawed research methodologies, "fairly strong" evidence exists to support acupressure for pain relief, specifically for menstrual pain, lower-back pain, and pain during childbirth. It has also been found to relieve chronic neck pain in women.[8] Research on acupressure for fibromyalgia symptoms has been inconclusive. Despite patient reports and some studies indicating that acupressure relieves headaches and painful arthritis, evidence for headache and other types of pain was found to be lacking.[9]

Acupressure can be self-performed to relieve tension and anxiety. Several acupressurists have posted how-to videos on YouTube, and various charts are available showing which pressure points correspond to different conditions. It is a good idea to have at least one session with a qualified practitioner who can demonstrate where to apply pressure and how much pressure to apply before you try it on your own.

Other Energy-Based Therapies

Japanese *Reiki* is a type of massage that is said to transfer energy from practitioner to patient. Like many other therapies, its pain-reducing quality may result from an ability to decrease tension. A Reiki master stimulates seven primary chakras, or energy fields, targeting different parts of the body that correspond to the area of discomfort: treatment for muscle pain would focus on the back, but it would concentrate on the head to treat fatigue. Limited research indicates that Reiki may help people with cancer, fibromyalgia, and other painful conditions. Other studies disagree.

Reflexology is said to improve circulation and reduce stress. Practitioners apply pressure to specific points on the feet that are believed to innervate different organs and muscle groups in the body: the arch of the foot represents the bladder, the ball of the foot represents the lung, and the base of the little toe corresponds to the ear. (Pressure may be applied instead to the hands or the ears.) In theory, manipulating these points stimulates nerve endings to increase circulation and generally improve function in the problem area. Despite the benefits of reflexology— it feels good and relieves cramping and tension in the feet—we have no evidence that it alleviates pain or improves health conditions.

Two other energy-based therapies are *Tui na,* a type of therapeutic massage that emphasizes rebalancing and restoration of the body's energy, and *Jin Shin Jyutsu,* which uses light pressure on specific body points to release tension and rebalance the body's energies.

Magnets

Magnets of varying sizes, shapes, and strengths are touted as miracle cures for arthritis, back pain, and most other conditions. Unlike the pulsed electromagnetic field therapy described in chapter 5, magnets sold for pain are static; their magnetic fields do not change. Magnetic pain cures in the form of copper bracelets, mattress pads, and shoe insoles are advertised to disrupt pain messages forwarded to the brain, yet no convincing scientific evidence supports these claims. Even though a clinical trial sponsored by the National Institutes of Health suggested a possible benefit for back pain with magnets, evidence of the safety and effectiveness of magnet therapy is scarce. Unless you have a pacemaker or an insulin pump, magnets appear to be safe when applied to the skin; they just do not seem to be effective. The prices of so-called pain-reducing magnets range from a few dollars to several hundred. Other forms of CAM may offer a better return on investment.

Mind-Body Movements

Yoga

Practiced regularly, *yoga* strengthens the body and comforts the mind. Performing low-impact movements with controlled breathing is a gentle and powerful way to increase blood supply to contracted muscles that limit a person's flexibility. Performed slowly and carefully, gentle yoga can help certain painful conditions. Not all poses will be possible for a body in pain, and some could be harmful. A well-trained instructor who has experience dealing with people in pain can explain proper alignment, adjust movements, and provide props to accommodate a sensitive wrist, back, knee, or neck. Yoga also has a positive effect on mental health, especially when it is combined with mindful meditation. This ancient physical and mental discipline is solely about the movement and the moment; it directs concentration to the present and teaches that we are more than our bodies and our pain.

Unlike many other CAM therapies, yoga's overall health benefits are well studied. It safely and effectively improves physical and psychological aspects of a chronically painful existence by ramping up energy and reducing negative feelings. A scholarly review of 81 studies concluded that "yoga interventions appeared to be equal or superior to exercise in nearly every outcome measured except those involving physical fitness."[10] Conclusive evidence is not available for yoga's impact on all pain conditions, but an NCCAM-sponsored study of 90 people with chronic low-back pain concluded that practicing Iyengar yoga reduced levels of disability, pain, and depression. In another trial involving 228 people with chronic back pain, patients who practiced yoga or conventional stretching exercises for 12 weeks experienced equally improved function and symptom improvement compared to those who used only a self-care book.[11] Other studies support yoga as a way to alleviate depression and the need for pain medication.[12]

Two well-designed studies show that yoga improves some of the physically and psychologically debilitating aspects of fibromyalgia. Patients in both projects showed greatly improved functionality, mood, and coping after eight weeks of yoga. In one study, 53 women had less continuous pain and fewer negative thoughts about their condition. They also had slightly elevated levels of *cortisol,* a hormone that heightens memory but also increases stress when secreted in high quantity, as it is during the body's fight-or-flight response. (Small increases of cortisol reduce sensitivity to pain.) Previous research suggests that women with fibromyalgia have lower-than-average cortisol levels, which contribute to pain, fatigue, and sensitivity to stress. The second study randomly placed 53 women who had been diagnosed with fibromyalgia for at least one year in two groups. The first group received standard care, while the second participated in a comprehensive program that included yoga stretches, meditation, breathing exercises, yoga-based coping instructions, and group discussion during two 75-minute sessions each week. At the end of the study, women assigned to the yoga program had significantly less pain and fatigue and were better able to cope and accept pain compared to the nonyoga group.[13]

Tai Chi and Qigong

Other Asian exercise regimens subdue stress and offer health benefits. *Tai chi,* which is often called "moving meditation," and *qigong* are mind-body therapies evolved from martial arts. Both are becoming increasingly popular in the United States. Unlike demanding cardiovascular workouts or strength training, tai chi and qigong are thoughtful alternatives that bring new perspective and focus on improving posture, flexibility, and inner strength. The beauty of these Asian exercises is that they are slow, purposeful, and easily learned. Because the fluid movements are gentle on the joints, tai chi and qigong are often recommended for frail older adults to improve their balance and help to prevent falls. Practicing tai chi has been shown to enhance the immune system and reduce blood pressure.

Most research on these movements involves elderly people; other studies indicate the value of tai chi and qigong as pain therapy. An analysis of 67 peer-reviewed, randomized controlled trials in 13 countries between 1993 and 2007 found sufficient evidence to suggest that tai chi and qigong produce a variety of health benefits and represent viable alternatives to conventional forms of exercise.[14] Tai chi is especially helpful as an adjunct therapy for people who have fibromyalgia or rheumatoid arthritis, for whom the slightest movement is often difficult. Compared to a control group of fibromyalgia patients who received wellness education and practiced stretching exercises, fibromyalgia patients who practiced tai chi for 12 weeks showed significantly improved sleep, mood, and quality of life. They retained those benefits after 24 weeks. People with rheumatoid arthritis reported worthwhile improvement of pain, mobility, and overall physical functionality after twice-weekly sessions for 12 weeks.[15] A different review of five randomized clinical trials of tai chi for patients with osteoarthritis in the knee found conflicting results. Two studies concluded that it improved pain and physical function more effectively than routine treatment; the other three studies did not.[16]

TAI CHI FOR FIBROMYALGIA

AT AGE 32, ELLEN WAS 40 POUNDS OVERWEIGHT and stressed from her job at a public relations firm. She avoided movement as much as possible because of a constant aching and stiffness in her arms, legs, neck, and back. Ellen had lived with fibromyalgia long enough to understand how difficult it is to treat. She was receptive, though surprised, when her doctor told her about a study showing that fibromyalgia patients who performed tai chi had relieved pain and fatigue. Ellen was not sure she would be able to perform the movements. She was skeptical of nontraditional exercise, and sometimes even the slightest movement made her muscle pain worse. But she was willing to try, so Ellen enrolled in a tai chi class at her local YWCA. She explained her condition to the instructor, who assessed Ellen's balance and flexibility and demonstrated the basic movements and breathing techniques.

For Ellen, tai chi was an easy, self-paced way to get her body moving again. She began by carefully practicing the low-impact movements for 10 to 15 minutes, gradually building up to one-hour sessions twice a week. On the days when she did not attend class, Ellen performed tai chi to a DVD at home. When she felt less motivated or less able, she still tried to keep up with her tai chi, focusing on the rhythmic movements and breathing, even if she needed to move more slowly. Ellen left class feeling calm and relaxed. Her sleep patterns improved, and she felt more energetic and more confident in her ability. After several weeks, her pain and other symptoms were noticeably better. She needed medication less frequently and in smaller doses.

Other Movement Therapies

Pilates emphasizes the quality of movement rather than the number of repetitions. Smooth, controlled movements are performed on a floor mat or with special equipment, focusing on breathing and holding correct spinal and pelvic alignment. Unlike exercises that work individual muscles,

Pilates works the entire body to strengthen core muscles and promote awareness of posture to lessen spinal stress and tension. A study by the University of Melbourne assigned patients with chronic low-back pain to two groups: one group performed an individualized Pilates regimen devised by a physical therapist; the other group performed a routine of generic back exercises. All participants attended supervised hourly sessions twice weekly. After 6 weeks, both groups reported significantly improved pain, functionality, and quality of life. The effects were also similar at 12 and 24 weeks, regardless of the type of exercise.[17] From this study, it appears that Pilates is no better or worse than standard back exercises.

Trager Psychophysical Integration sessions include passive and active components. During table work sessions, a practitioner uses his hands to isolate and gently manipulate joints, muscles, and fascia. These sessions are reinforced by more active "Mentastics," free-form dancelike movements performed at home or in a group setting. The movements are intended to decrease tension by recalling the feeling of deep relaxation. Very little research on this therapy exists. A limited study found that it relieved shoulder pain in patients with spinal cord injury as effectively as acupuncture.[18]

Feldenkrais is said to produce higher levels of physical and mental prowess by concentrating on the relationship between movement and thought. The goal of Feldenkrais is somewhat unique, since it concentrates on neuromuscular reeducation brought about by self-awareness. Hands-on sessions conducted by a Functional Integration practitioner are intended to detect minute resistance in movement patterns that can represent physical, emotional, or psychological limitations. During Awareness through Movement group sessions, participants are verbally guided through a carefully designed sequence of movements. In a small Swedish study, women with neck and shoulder pain reported positive experiences from Feldenkrais treatment, even though they considered the self-performed exercises to be difficult.[19]

Holistic and Nature-Based Therapies

People have used herbs and botanicals to treat physical ailments since the beginning of recorded time, and probably long before. Americans who are looking for ways to improve their health and find relief from pain spend billions of dollars each year on herbs and nutritional supplements. Some practitioners eschew modern treatments and synthetic drugs (even synthetic versions of a plant's active ingredient), depending instead on the curative properties of teas, dried leaves, and plant extracts. Some of these methodologies have been handed down over generations.

Herbs and Nutritional Supplements

Plants have traditionally formed the basis of our pharmacopeia, and people like the idea of trying to improve their health or relieve pain by taking substances that they consider to be natural and harmless. Truthfully, compounds in commercial herbal products are often anything but natural, and some herbs may magnify the effect or otherwise interfere with medications and produce unwanted side effects. Dietary supplements and herbal products, even those labeled "natural," are not required to undergo the rigorous testing and approval process used for prescription drugs. Manufacturers are responsible for ensuring that their products are safe and honestly marketed. Without sufficient government scrutiny or guidelines for standardization, some preparations are not what they appear to be. Contamination from animal products has been found in many products, and the ingredients often do not match labeling information. Numerous government warnings and legal actions have targeted unsafe products and vendors who make misleading or false statements about their products. Current law allows labels of dietary supplements, including herbs, to claim that the product improves health in some way if research (any research) supports the claim. Labels must also include this text: "This statement has not been evaluated by the U.S. Food and Drug Administration (FDA). This product is not intended to diagnose, treat, cure, or prevent any disease."

Herbs have been used as a pain remedy in much of the world for thousands of years, but in most cases, they are poorly studied and lack convincing scientific evidence. Limited studies of painful conditions in humans (rather than laboratory animals) show that some herbs and nutritional supplements, including the following, may be beneficial for pain. More credible research is needed.

- Acetyl-L-carnitine (ALC) shows promise for diabetic peripheral neuropathy. Two 52-week double-blind, placebo-controlled studies involving 1,257 people evaluated the benefit of taking 500 mg or 1,000 mg daily. Individuals who took ALC, especially those who took the higher dosage, had improved levels of pain and sensory perception. The supplement also appeared to promote nerve-fiber regeneration.[20]
- Arnica montana gel may be as effective as gels containing ibuprofen, according to studies of individuals with osteoarthritis of the knee or hand.[21]
- Devil's claw has a long history of use as an anti-inflammatory and an analgesic. In randomized controlled trials, the African plant showed promise for alleviating acute back pain as effectively as NSAIDs and a COX-2 inhibitor, although it can cause gastrointestinal discomfort. Other studies indicate that taking devil's claw extract for at least four weeks may moderately relieve osteoarthritis symptoms and reduce the amount of pain medication needed, compared to taking a placebo.[22]
- Feverfew, also known as wild chamomile, is related to sunflowers. It contains parthenolide, a compound known to lessen inflammation and decrease constriction of blood vessels. Even though some research found no benefit in feverfew compared to a placebo, several studies have suggested that it may be a viable treatment for migraine headaches. It has properties similar to those of COX-2 inhibitors, so there is concern about its long-term effect, especially for people with coronary disease.
- Ginger is known to aid digestion and decrease nausea; evidence of its analgesic properties remains inconclusive. It does appear to reduce inflammation in animals; whether that benefit applies consistently to humans remains to be seen. Among patients with osteoarthritis of the knee or hip who participated in a Russian experiment, 21 men and women who took daily doses of ginger and glucosamine fared better than 22 others who took a common osteoarthritis medication (diclofenac) and glucosamine during the same period. Both groups showed decreased inflammation and

pain; the ginger group had significantly less gastrointestinal disturbance.[23]

- Glucosamine with or without chondroitin is one of the most popular supplements sold. As described in chapter 2, multiple studies have examined its effectiveness for arthritis, with mixed results. The most comprehensive investigation, the Glucosamine/Chondroitin Arthritis Intervention Trial (GAIT), found that glucosamine or chondroitin taken alone did not relieve osteoarthritis knee pain more effectively than a placebo. Taken in combination, the supplements were somewhat effective for moderate to severe pain—they did not benefit individuals with mild pain.

- Avocado-soy unsaponifiables, which are extracts made from avocado and soybean oils, have been used as anti-inflammatories in Europe for years. Supportive European studies are encouraging for these extracts as treatments for knee and hip arthritis. Researchers suspect that the extract decreases the body's production of inflammatory neurochemicals, thereby protecting cartilage from breaking down.

- Numerous studies are investigating the analgesic properties of turmeric, the spice that gives curry powder its characteristic yellow hue. Most research has concentrated on curcumin, an active ingredient in turmeric that reduces inflammation and helps to reduce symptoms of irritable bowel syndrome and arthritis. Curcumin is known to interfere with some types of chemotherapy and blood thinners.

- Gamma linolenic acid (GLA) is an omega-6 fatty acid from evening primrose and black currant seed oils. Popularly used for premenstrual and menopausal symptoms, it may, according to preliminary evidence, somewhat curtail symptoms of inflammatory conditions, including rheumatoid arthritis and diabetic neuropathy.[24] Unlike most other omega-6 fatty acids, which promote inflammation, GLA may actually reduce it. Omega-3 fatty acids are more potent anti-inflammatories.

- Beneficial probiotic microbes may help people who suffer from irritable bowel syndrome, gastritis, and other painful digestive conditions, especially those that cause nausea and diarrhea.[25]

Some probiotics may also have anti-inflammatory properties. Healthy bowels and digestive systems have trillions of microorganisms that keep harmful bacteria in check and boost absorption of nutrients. Ingesting foods or supplements with live probiotics can help replace healthy levels of "good" intestinal bacteria that are sometimes diminished by inflammation, antibiotics, and other medications. Yogurt and kefir (a fermented milk drink made with grain) are among the best sources of natural probiotics. Read the product labels: you are looking for a product that lists "live, active cultures" as an ingredient. More research is needed to identify which strains of probiotics might be best for certain conditions.

- At the University of Maryland, rats with induced arthritis had symptom relief when they were given a version of Huo Luo Xiao Ling Dan (HLXL), a classic herb combination that is often used in traditional Chinese medicine.[26]

Information about herbs and supplements can be found at the websites of the National Center for Complementary and Alternative Medicine (nccam.nih.gov), the Memorial Sloan-Kettering Cancer Center (www.mskcc.org/cancer-care/integrative-medicine/about-herbs), and the Food and Drug Administration (www.fda.gov). All of these websites provide information about the safety and efficacy of herbs and dietary supplements. Research assessments and product reviews by Consumer Labs (www.consumerlabs.com) and the National Standard Research Collaboration (www.nationalstandard.com) are more extensive and are available with a subscription.

Aromatherapy

Lying in a warm bath scented with aromatic oils, enjoying an *aromatherapy* massage, or inhaling essential oil from a handkerchief are easy ways to unwind from the pressures of a painful day. Plant oils have been a mainstay in the healing practices of different cultures for centuries. Archaeological discoveries show that ancient Egyptians used essential oils as sedatives and analgesics, and the Bible tells of using infused oils as remedies for various ailments. Despite bold marketing claims that aromatherapy relieves pain and even increases cognitive function, its primary benefit is the ability to calm and relax.

Aromatherapists maintain that essential oils work by stimulating areas of the brain that regulate emotion and long-term memory. Another hypothesis is that olfactory sensors in the nose influence certain mood-modulating neurotransmitters in the emotional centers of the brain. Some proponents theorize that essential oils work by interacting with hormones and enzymes in the blood. From practical experience, everyone is familiar with the pleasant feeling of inhaling an enticing odor. The aroma of baking bread, freshly brewed coffee, or fragrant flowers is enough to make many people smile. In theory, that is how aromatherapy produces a direct nose-to-brain effect; our reactions to odors and aromas are partially based in memory. Vanilla is one of the most popular aromas, perhaps because we associate it with warmth, happiness, and comfort. It will not have the same tantalizing effect if it makes you nauseous or brings back unpleasant memories. An informal study at the Memorial Sloan-Kettering Cancer Center tested the effects of five fragrances on 85 patients before they had an MRI scan. By far, patients responded more favorably to a vanilla-like aroma—63 percent said it made them feel less anxious about the claustrophobic effects of MRI. Another project at the Smell and Taste Treatment and Research Foundation (www.smellandtaste.org) underscores this premise. Among 50 migraine patients who used penlike devices scented with a green-apple fragrance at the onset of their headaches, 15 who liked the odor experienced a significant reduction in the severity of their headache. The 35 subjects who disliked the odor had no improvement in their symptoms.[27]

The only large randomized controlled study of aromatherapy was funded by NCCAM and conducted at Ohio State University. Researchers measured the effect of lavender oil (which is said to have a relaxing effect) and lemon oil (associated with uplifted mood) on healing, mood, immune function, heart rate, and blood pressure. Fifty-six volunteers participated, including some who were proponents of aromatherapy; others had no opinion one way or the other. When the results were tallied, neither smell had any significant positive physiological effect; participants who smelled the lemon oil said they felt somewhat happier.[28]

Despite studies of aromatherapy that have produced inconsistent and inconclusive data, some evidence suggests that inhaling the vapors of peppermint or ginger essential oils reduces symptoms of nausea and vomiting.[29] Some hospitals provide aromatherapy with rose and lavender oil to help pregnant women felt less anxious and fearful about delivery.

Check with your doctor before trying aromatherapy. It is generally considered to be safe, although certain types of essential oils are not recommended during pregnancy or for women who have estrogen-positive breast cancers. In some people, certain oils may cause headache, nausea, or an allergic reaction. Read labels when purchasing aromatherapy products to be sure that they contain essential oils—thousands of cosmetics, toiletries, and candles sold as "aromatherapy" contain only synthetic fragrances that do not have the same properties as essential oils. Essential oils used in aromatherapy are diluted; rubbing undiluted oils directly into the skin can cause irritation. Nor should they be ingested. Experimenting with different essential oils might help you determine which one, if any, makes you feel better. There is nothing wrong with feeling more relaxed, as long as you do not expect aromatherapy to eliminate your pain or heal health conditions.

Homeopathy

Homeopathic remedies are said to improve health by hormesis, meaning they produce a beneficial effect with low-dose substances that would be toxic or lethal in greater quantity. The same principle is behind vaccines or inoculations, which introduce small doses of harmful pathogens to stimulate the production of helpful antibodies. Homeopathic ointments, gels, creams, and tablets are made from natural substances from plants, minerals, or metals. The FDA identifies active ingredients (and their strength and purity) that may be included in homeopathic preparations; the agency does not evaluate products for effectiveness or safety. Homeopathic products do not always include all of the ingredients listed on the label, and some are so diluted that almost no trace of the original substance remains. It is difficult to explain how something with almost no active ingredient might improve or heal any condition. Researching homeopathic medicine is challenging, because no prescribing standards of dilutions exist, and treatments are customized for individuals; several people with the same condition might have different homeopathic treatments. No well-controlled, good-quality studies substantiate homeopathy as an effective treatment for chronic pain or any other specific condition, yet it is quite popular throughout the world.

Naturopathy

Naturopathic medicine (also called *naturopathy*) is a holistic system based on the healing powers of nature to restore health and prevent disease. Modern practitioners use a combination of noninvasive approaches to stimulate the body's ability to heal itself. Treatment might include herbs, massage, acupuncture, lifestyle changes, advice about nutrition, and a variety of other traditional and contemporary therapies.

Ayurveda

Ayurvedic medicine is thought to be the world's oldest healing system. Practiced in India for more than 5,000 years, it is a holistic approach to physical, emotional, and spiritual health. This ancient practice teaches that disease begins when we live out of harmony with our internal and external nature. The fundamental principle of Ayurvedic treatment is that we are a combination of five "doshas," or universal elements: air, fire, water, earth, and ether. When balanced, these elements support health and well-being. Illness and pain are believed to develop when physical, emotional, or spiritual energies become unbalanced. Treatment may involve a customized regimen of exercise, meditation, diet, and herbal preparations that are intended to rebalance the troubled dosha to restore harmony in mind, body, and spirit.

Interest in Ayurvedic medicine is growing in the United States, and even though scientific studies have not validated its effectiveness as a whole, some components are known to benefit stress and inflammation and positively affect overall health. An Ayurvedic "prescription" for some conditions, for example, might include a vegetarian diet, which is known to be heart-healthy. A first-of-its kind, double-blind, randomized controlled 36-week study of rheumatoid arthritis patients at the University of California–Los Angeles compared a classic Ayurvedic regimen to methotrexate (a commonly used medication for rheumatoid arthritis) alone and a combination of Ayurvedic medicine and methotrexate. All three treatments produced similar results, but patients who were treated with the Ayurvedic regimen had fewer adverse events.[30]

Much more study is required, yet small trials of some Ayurvedic herbs have produced compelling conclusions. A mixture of these herbs was shown to relieve constipation from analgesics as effectively as standard laxatives, and *mucuna pruriens,* another herb used by Ayurvedic practitioners, shows promise. Scientists are researching other Ayurvedic herbs to determine whether their active ingredients might help to treat symptoms of Alzheimer's disease, anxiety, Parkinson's disease, and side effects from chemotherapy. One concern about Ayurvedic herbal mixtures is that some of them include toxic metals and minerals. An NCCAM-funded investigation in 2008 found that one in five Ayurvedic medicines manufactured in India and the United States and sold on the Internet contained lead, mercury, and arsenic in greater quantities than are considered to be safe. Some individuals have developed lead poisoning after ingesting these preparations.[31]

A final note, about paying for CAM. Most patients pay out-of-pocket for CAM therapies, yet health care insurance often covers the cost of acupuncture, yoga, and certain other CAM therapies when they are recommended by a physician to improve a specific health condition. Some health insurers do not pay for CAM services but negotiate with certain providers for discounted rates for their members.

SUMMARY POINTS

- **Complementary and alternative medicines are tools that may relieve symptoms but should not replace conventional pain-management strategies.**
- **Few CAM therapies have been thoroughly researched for safety and effectiveness.**
- **Talk to your physician before beginning any CAM therapies, to ensure that they will not cause harmful side effects or interfere with your treatment and medications.**
- **Review the credentials and experience of CAM practitioners and providers before engaging their services.**

Spirit over Pain

Each of us is more than body and mind. We are also spiritual beings. Spiritual health—the comfort, peace, and significance we find in life—is as essential to our well-being as physical and emotional balance. Increasingly, health care professionals and pain experts are recognizing that chronic pain is an amalgam of physical, emotional, and spiritual influences, and that a comprehensive approach to reduce suffering must address all three. Nevertheless, the role of spirituality in health care is still controversial, and it is a topic that many practitioners do not feel comfortable discussing.

The various members of your health care team are important partners in managing your chronic pain, but you are the captain of your spiritual ship. You are the one who can harness your spiritual awareness and power to make life with chronic pain not only bearable but meaningful and productive as well. You may find that meaning in a religious service surrounded by others or as you meditate in your own home. What is most important is not where you find it but that you find it. Chronic pain by its nature is incurable, yet you can heal your damaged or broken spirit and regain a deep and lasting sense of happiness and comfort. The spiritual coping strategies described in this chapter work by shifting the perception of pain. You feel more pain when you are resentful or depressed and less when you are content with your life.

Virtually everyone who suffers from chronic pain long enough eventually faces a crisis of spirit. Grief, heartache, and loss—all common by-products of chronic pain—test the personal core beliefs that ordinarily define our spiritual substance and help us cope with life's struggles. Such is the case with prolonged pain. Living with it can be an endless cycle of spiritual frustration: the more you become dispirited and disillusioned, and the more you lose faith, the more pain and suffering you feel. You may grieve for the functionality that pain steals away or feel robbed of hope and not know how to get it back. But such experiences can teach us what is truly important in life. This doesn't mean you should ignore or resist pain or stoically endure it. But you can acknowledge it and re-affirm your spiritual strength to limit the impact of pain on your life.

Religion, Spirituality, or Both?

What, exactly, is spirituality? It cannot be seen or measured; yet spirituality is a vital part of the human experience. It is a state of mind, the concept that there is more to life than what we experience with our five senses, and the deeply personal connection we feel to a presence that is greater than us. For most Americans, that means God. For others, it might be a universal consciousness or a personal conviction that life should be lived in a deliberate and purposeful way.

Spirituality can also be defined as a process in which we seek to:

- understand the value of life
- come to know our true selves
- discover our individual place in the world and how we fit in
- feel connected to others
- pursue personal growth throughout our lives

Your spiritual perspective is influenced by your religious, philosophical, and cultural assumptions. While many people consider religion and spirituality to be one and the same, they are different. Someone who is religious subscribes to the core beliefs and practices of an organized and usually ancient faith system: Eastern religions such as Buddhism, Taoism, and Hinduism, and Western religions that are based on an omnipotent God, including Judaism, Christianity, and Islam. Spirituality defines our individual beliefs: the truths we live by, though not necessarily according to religious theory. You may be religious but lack spirituality. (Hopefully, most religious people are also spiritual!) Conversely, you may be deeply spiritual without the structure of organized religion, believing that moral, loving behavior makes the world a better place. Or you might consider yourself to be both religious and spiritual. Whether you are deeply religious or strongly spiritual, your values provide your life's spiritual anchor. When pain makes you question your own faith, you may feel that that anchor is lost, and you may give up all hope of ever again living a normal life. Spiritual strength can help you cope with your pain, learn how to restore a sense of direction in your life, and transcend the physical experience.

A survey of 920 patients found that most of them believed their physicians would be more understanding and compassionate during office visits if they understood their patients' spiritual beliefs:[1]

- 87 percent wanted their doctors to understand how their beliefs helped them deal with being sick.
- 85 percent believed their doctors would understand them better.
- 62 percent would welcome a discussion of spirituality if they suffered from chronic pain.
- People aged 30 to 64 most welcomed spiritual discussions.
- Women were more likely than men to change their medical treatment based on spirituality.

A different study of hospitalized patients' views about religious and spiritual concerns identified similar beliefs:[2]

- 41 percent desired a discussion of their religious and spiritual concerns while hospitalized.
- 32 percent of inpatients reported having a discussion of their concerns.
- Religious patients and those experiencing severe pain were more likely to have these discussions.
- Patients who discussed their spirituality were more likely to rate their care at the highest level.

Pain and Suffering Are Not the Same

Among the millions of people who live with debilitating chronic pain, what is the difference between those who have limited, unhappy lives and others who are content and productive despite their condition? The real difference is that some people are able to limit the level of control that pain has in their lives. They more often depend on their spiritual resources to cope. Many credit spirituality as the vital force that helps them make sense of their pain and keeps them moving past it. More than 60 percent of people with pain pray to deal with chronic pain, and up to 40 percent report becoming more religious or spiritual because of it.[3]

Pain and suffering may seem to be one and the same, but they are quite different. Pain is the unpleasant physical symptom of something gone wrong in your body. Suffering is a by-product of the conscious or subconscious meaning that you assign to your pain. While the temporary quality of acute pain rarely requires spiritual fortitude, chronic pain challenges you to respond more profoundly; the nature of your response determines your level of suffering.

You can change how you react to pain and minimize the suffering it causes, even though eliminating it may be beyond your control. You probably cannot will your pain away, but changing what you believe about it is the next best thing. Consider a man in his twenties who breaks a leg while skiing. He takes pain medication, hobbles around in a cast for a couple of months, and then recovers fully and returns to his normal functionality and routine. Now imagine that the same man falls and breaks the same leg 30 years later because of a bone tumor. Compared to his earlier fracture, even if the amount of tissue damage and nerve signals are identical, this time he will probably experience more suffering because he has much more at stake: a questionable future that might include disability, compromised financial status, and many other life-affecting issues. Thus he will worry, stress, and focus on the pain much more than he did many years before. He will suffer more not because of the pain, which is no more or less than it was previously, but because of his reaction to it.

Pain leads to different destinations. Left spiritually unattended, it can direct you to protracted anxiety and suffering, spreading like a crack across a windshield until it affects more and more of your life. But pain can also guide you along a more fulfilling path of appreciation, acceptance, and growth, helping you to become stronger than you ever were before. You have a choice: suffer with chronic pain or choose not to. As Zen wisdom dictates, pain is inevitable. Suffering is optional.

Does Pain Have Meaning?

Many of us move through life in a blur. Caught up in the hectic pace of the modern world, we rarely think about the bigger spiritual picture until a jarring incident—a tragic accident or the death of a loved one—jolts us into questioning our place in life or the very issue of our existence. Chronic pain is such an experience. It drags us from our spiritual comfort zone to a confusing spiritual crossroads. Cut off from your work and your passions, estranged from family and friends, you may become spiritually isolated by chronic pain at its worst. Are you alone? Is God or a greater power with you? Are you destined to be lost in your pain for the remainder of your life?

Depending on your religious perspective, you may believe your pain has a purpose, and inevitably you will wonder whether it also has meaning: is it your destiny or a part of God's plan for you? When you see that others around you are not afflicted with chronic pain, you might ask, Why, then, am I? If you feel victimized by your pain, you are not alone. The "Why me?" question is common among individuals who live with pain. No answer improves the situation. Thinking and rethinking it brings no benefit and creates angst that only intensifies the pain. "Why me?" is more an expression of spiritual pain than a question expecting an answer. A better question is "What now?" How do you find purpose in your pain and perfect what you can add to yourself and to the world? Does your chronic condition present a silver lining that can help you grow spiritually and improve your relationships with God and with others? When you can transform your suffering and use it for personal growth, you will feel better, cope better, and limit the control pain holds over your life.

Pain as Punishment

You may hold God or the devil responsible, or you may even consider your pain itself to be a force with evil intent. Perhaps you wonder how God can allow so much suffering in the world, including the pain you continue to feel. The concept of pain as punishment is rooted in the Judeo-Christian belief that it is a kind of divine payback for our sins. (The word *pain* is derived from the Latin word *poena*, meaning a fine or a penalty.) Islam, Buddhism, and Hinduism believe that pain is part of karma, punishment for moral misdeeds in a previous life. Some religions teach that suffering is actually a kindness from God and that suffering in this life diminishes the need for a person to suffer in eternal life after death. These beliefs can trigger feelings of relief, understanding, or guilt. Guilt has bad connotations, but it is an emotion that if used properly can lead to personal growth and improvement; if used improperly, it can lead to increased depression.

Pain as Education

Many religions view pain and suffering as educational rather than punitive, as a method God uses to help us understand some divine principle, similar to the way parents use discipline to teach their children. If you consider God to be good and loving, and you believe that he is using pain as an instrument to test or educate you, then there must be some reason for it: a reminder of weakness, a lesson in humility, or an impetus to draw closer to him. (This same rationale applies to the universe or a higher power if you do not believe in God.) Such a belief also makes it easier to accept that your pain must have some positive component that you may not understand. People who believe in a benevolent God and use religious or spiritual strategies to cope with life issues generally have a better sense of self and quality of life than those who view the world pessimistically and struggle with meaning in their lives.[4]

Most of us tend to think of pain as a tremendous hardship without redeeming value, but it is healthier to think of pain as an educational tool that helps us to grow spiritually, to extend our relationship with a higher power, and to increase our compassion for others. Pain can be a fire sent to temper our strength and a tool to help us achieve spiritual goals. As the German philosopher Friedrich Nietzsche wrote in 1888, "That which does not kill me makes me stronger." Many experiences in this world, including chronic conditions, can be painful, but they do not need to bring about spiritual hardship.

Seven Spiritual Tools to Help You Move beyond Pain

Persistent pain robs you of the best part of your life by laying claim to your consciousness. All-consuming pain constricts your view of the world. It shrinks your ability to function and your outlook on life and limits your relationships until you feel broken, isolated, and alone. Religious and spiritual theologies frequently include the concept of transcendence, the ability to rise above physical, emotional, or spiritual pain. The idea that we can be more than our physical experience can be particularly appealing when that physical existence is unpleasant. Transcending pain is a process. Using a variety of spiritual tools, you can rise above your suffering so that you restore joy to your life and live an expanded existence even when your pain continues.

1. Reframing Spiritual Thoughts

Applying the reframing methods discussed in chapter 4 to spiritual concepts can change the way you think and help you to move beyond your pain. Start by becoming aware of the negative spiritual impact your pain seems to have on your thoughts; then replace the negative thoughts with spiritually affirming thoughts. Your pain will interfere less with your life when your thinking is more like "Even with pain there is much to be

TABLE 7.1 Reframing spiritual thoughts

Thoughts that make pain worse	Thoughts that limit pain's impact
My pain is punishment	Pain is a wakeup call: I am mortal; it is time to change
God doesn't like me	Pain can help me become more empathetic and caring
Why is this happening to me?	Pain can help me recognize the empathy and caring of others
Pain has no meaning or value	Pain can help me see the hand of a higher intelligence or God in my life
	I can view pain as a way to learn about my strengths and my ability to overcome
	Pain can open me to the help of others
	Pain can open me to the help of God or a higher power

thankful for," rather than "My life is ruined," "I'll never get over this pain," or "Why is God abandoning me?" Another way to gain power over your pain is to appreciate it (table 7.1). By reframing the negative spiritual worth you have assigned to your pain and focusing instead on the goodness your life holds and the good that you can still do, you limit pain's influence in your life.

2. Motivation to Engage Life

Presented with a pain-treatment plan, people often ask what level of relief they can expect. Most understand that their pain will not be eliminated, even though they still hope that it will be. Managing your pain keeps it from running or ruining your life and gives you the best possible future. But to cooperate with the plan, you must give up the expectation that your life is never going to get better or, alternatively, that it will somehow get better on its own and miraculously return to the way it used to be.

Focus on where you can make a difference, rather than where you cannot. You have little command over the damage your body experiences, but you have considerable control over attitudes that influence your reaction to pain. Learn to let go of feelings of self-pity, victimization, and martyrdom. You may feel that your pain is a result of life treating you

Noted psychologist Victor Frankl lost his father, mother, brother, and wife to the Holocaust, but he himself survived four Nazi death camps, including Auschwitz. Suffering from hunger and cold and expecting death, Frankl exercised his most important freedom, to determine his own attitude and spiritual health, despite the misery of the camps and the sadistic actions of the guards. He did this by thinking of his wife, imagining her face, her laughter, and her voice. This mental exercise strengthened his will to survive when so many around him gave up hope and died. Asked why he wrote *Man's Search for Meaning* after the war, Frankl replied, "I had wanted simply to convey to the reader by way of concrete example that life holds a potential meaning under any conditions, even the most miserable ones." In his book, Frankl wrote, "[Concentration camp survivors] offer sufficient proof that everything can be taken from a man but one thing: the last of his freedoms—to choose one's attitude in any given set of circumstances, to choose one's own way." He also said, "Man is not destroyed by suffering; he is destroyed by suffering without meaning."

unfairly or that it is something you do not deserve. As self-help author Dennis Wholey said, "Chronic pain is not fair, but expecting life to always treat us fairly because we are good people is like expecting a bull not to gore us because we are vegetarians." Replace your feelings of helplessness with positive feelings that enhance your spiritual strength. Your pain may keep you from some things in life—your desire to be a runner or to work at your chosen career, or your ability to frolic with your children (or grandchildren), but those limitations need not keep you from a full and meaningful life or separate you from happiness. Downgrade your pain from an impasse to a bump on the road.

3. Prayer

Prayer is the most common non-pharmaceutical method of pain management and the most popular form of alternative medicine practiced in the United States.[5] Data released by the American Psychological Association show that the number of adults in the United States who pray for their health increased 36 percent between 1999 and 2007 (these people said they prayed to supplement the benefits of their health care, not to replace their health care).[6] More than half of the 1,204 respondents to a nationwide poll conducted by ABC News, *USA Today*, and the Stanford University Medical Center said they use prayer against pain—90 percent said it "worked well" and 51 percent said it worked "very well."[7] Numerous other studies have come to similar conclusions, finding that people with chronic pain frequently rely on religious activities or beliefs, including prayer, to help them cope.

Prayer is a conversation between you and a greater-than-human intelligence, a heartfelt conversation that requires no special skills or experience. The concept can be difficult if you have no religious background. You might wonder, What is this all about, or What is the point? If God (or some other universal intelligence) is all-powerful and all-knowing, why should you try to tell him about your pain or remind him how great he is? If God gave pain to you, who are you to ask that he take it back? These are valid questions. Prayer, however, is not for God's sake. It is for yours. The power of prayer, performed silently or aloud, is the profound feelings it arouses within us: a sense of connection with a divine presence that consoles us with serenity and a hopeful perspective. Through prayer we release control of our pain to a higher power, and in doing so we relieve ourselves of the burden of pain and the stress it causes. The result is more positive feelings and an improved sense of contentment.

THE POWER OF PRAYER

Brian Sternberg was the world's best pole vaulter until a trampoline accident in 1963 left him quadriplegic. Soon afterward, he was living with nerve pain throughout his body and was deeply depressed. Then he turned to prayer. In a *Look* magazine article a year after his accident, he said, "Having faith is a necessary step toward one of two things. Being healed is one of them. Peace of mind, if healing doesn't come, is the other. Either will suffice."

TABLE 7.2 Getting started with prayer

Prayer does not need to be	Prayer can be
Complicated	Said simply, as if you were speaking with another person
Said aloud	Said silently or aloud
Performed in church	Performed anywhere
Of a certain length	Short or long
Only for the deeply faithful	Beneficial for anyone
Said in a certain way	Different things to different people
Scheduled	Done at any time

If you think of prayer as a type of meditation, it is easy to understand why it calms and uplifts the spirit in the same way meditation does. Both actions promote a consciousness of hope that lowers stress and blood pressure. The process may be different—meditating is an inward concentration, while praying is an outward appeal to a greater being—but the mind-body-spirit benefit is the same. Whether your prayers are short and to the point or lengthy and detailed, prayer serves best when it is genuine and expressed humbly and from the heart (table 7.2). Prayer changes us. It makes us more humble, more grateful, and spiritually stronger, whether we pray to God, the universe, or a higher power. Prayer may or may not eliminate pain, but it is fine to believe in an improved outlook and even hope for a miracle.

Some people wonder whether prayer can backfire. Prayer can bring about a less-than-desirable effect, especially if we view it as a demand of God; in that case, frustration and increased suffering may result from unanswered appeals. It is best to see prayer as an opportunity to work on ourselves and on our relationship with God.

4. Spiritual Meditation

Mindfulness and other forms of secular meditation shut out external factors that cause stress and intensify pain. Spiritual meditation produces a similar effect in a different way. It directs the mind to a spiritual ideal, rather than to our inner consciousness. While meditation is helpful in various aspects of our lives, spiritual meditation helps us to understand and appreciate the positive forces in life. It focuses our thoughts toward harmony, happiness, and peace as it builds a focused path to a higher intelligence so that we are better equipped to master life's trials and tribulations. Spiritual awareness and strength enable you to live through your pain as you carry on with your life.

Unlike prayer, which is a conversation with the divine and a plea for help, spiritual meditation opens you to the greater universe and directs the power of your own mind toward self-healing. This form of enormously beneficial meditation involves repeating spiritually relevant words. A 2008 study of individuals with vascular headaches concluded that participants who repeated spiritually significant phrases felt an increased presence of love and comfort, which translated into improved pain tolerance. Participants who repeated "God is peace," "God is good," "God is joy," or "God is love" for 20 minutes daily for one month experienced significantly reduced frequency and intensity of headaches and much improved spiritual happiness and overall quality of life.[8] In another study, individuals who practiced spiritual meditation daily for two weeks tolerated more pain for longer periods and were less anxious about pain than others who practiced secular meditation. Research involving migraine patients produced similar results.[9]

Regular spiritual meditation can restore and maintain spiritual balance, so you become less judgmental of your pain and assign it less meaning. Through meditation, you can reduce your anticipation and negative appraisal of pain. The pain will still be there, but you can move away from it by creating a life that is full, productive, and joyful. It's usually helpful to have some assistance in getting started with meditation. You can search

FINDING SPIRITUAL RELIEF WITH MEDITATION

1. Sit comfortably with your back supported and your eyes closed.
2. Consciously relax all your muscles one by one, from head to toe.
3. Breathe through your nose, keeping your mouth closed.
4. Focus on the inhalation and exhalation of your breath.
5. Concentrate on a mantra as you inhale.*
6. Feel the intent of the words you say.
7. Repeat the words as you exhale.
8. Continue to breathe slowly, focusing on the words.
9. If your mind wanders, return your focus to your breath.
10. Open yourself to feelings of love, comfort, and belonging.
11. Practice once or twice daily for at least 5 minutes (10 minutes is better).

*Spoken silently or aloud, a mantra (one or more words repeated during meditation) directs your mind to a single point of focus. Whatever words you choose—"I am at peace," "joy," "God is love," or others—should be spiritually substantive to you.

online or in the telephone directory for a spiritual meditation class. Many books and DVDs are also available.

I meditate daily and pray often. I don't just pray for what I want, but also for what I and others already have. I often use Mindfulness Meditation with an emphasis on loving kindness, which is the desire to want someone, including ourself, to be happy. It's about cultivating positive emotion, which I love and keep with me throughout the day. Rather than focusing on what I've lost, I prefer to think about the gifts I continue to receive from my journey with pain: how much deeper my life, relationships, and work are as a result of my injury 30 years ago. The positive affirmations that I repeat to myself continue to bring me to a more peaceful place. I've never said good-bye to anything I love because that closes off the possibility of regaining it. I see people with pain doing this far too often; they decide that everything they love is gone forever because it's gone now. But I'm living proof that not only can we reinvent ourselves to find different ways of living our passions, but many of them eventually come back.

—Cynthia

TABLE 7.3   Examples of spiritually satisfying rituals

Personal rituals	Rituals involving others
Meditating	Attending religious services or retreats
Praying	Participating in a prayer group
Reading the Bible, Koran, or other inspirational material	Observing religious holidays
	Taking part in community service
Deep breathing	Participating in a pain support group
Journaling	Attending regular gatherings with others
Exercising	Observing traditions for and with your children
Spending time with pets	
Listening to spiritually satisfying music	Celebrating birthdays and anniversaries
	Singing in a choir

5. Rituals

Individual and group rituals remind us of life's value beyond the pace and pressure of ordinary life. Rituals can also be powerful tools that help us relax, reflect, and gain from our own inner spirit. Unlike a habit, which is something you do over and over without thinking, a ritual is a conscious and planned repetitive action that satisfies and comforts. Personal rituals can be simple and idiosyncratic: starting each morning with a cup of coffee or tea as you catch up on the mail, or relaxing each evening in a scented bath as you listen to soothing music. Many rituals are based in religion (table 7.3). They may also involve others, such as Sunday family dinners or observing the Sabbath. Spiritual rituals create a sense of continuity that helps to counteract existential crises.

Whether alone or with others, observing positive rituals is rewarding on many levels. Consider what you can do to restore your spiritual balance and remove yourself from pain. You may find that briefly walking the dog each morning as you focus on the pleasantness of your surroundings gives your day a new positive perspective. Often, chronic pain creates feelings of isolation; creating a ritual to deal with those feelings— attending a support group or prayer meeting, making a point of talking or e-mailing with a friend several times a week, or setting aside special times with your partner—will help you remain connected to others and maintain a sense of belonging.

6. Gratitude

The Roman philosopher Cicero called gratitude "the mother of all virtues." Modern science proves him right; it shows that being truly thankful not only is good manners but also is profoundly favorable to one's mental and physical health. Being grateful is like yoga for the spirit—it feels good. More importantly, it is a powerful motivator that leads to life transformations. Gratitude shifts your focus from what your life lacks to what it already has. It is a simple mental action that buffers against cynicism and negative emotions. It makes you happier, and that translates to better overall health.

Behavioral and psychological research and anecdotal reports show that people who are grateful tend to have less pain and more satisfaction with life. They are more resilient, cope better, and are generally happier than others who have a negative and constricted view of themselves and the world.[10] When you're grateful, it is hard to be anxious, depressed, or self-centered. And the more you focus on gratitude, the harder it is to focus on pain. This seems intuitive—we feel better when we are grateful than when we are not—yet it is easy to forget to be thankful, especially when we are in pain. Gratefulness in the midst of suffering begins with acceptance. In the case of chronic pain, that means accepting that pain exists in your life and that you may always have it to some degree. Let go of the notion that you should not have pain or do not deserve it. Determine instead that you will no longer let pain keep you from appreciating aspects of your life for which you can and should be thankful.

You are probably wondering how you can be grateful about pain, which disrupts so many facets of your life. You may not feel thankful for your migraine headaches, your back pain, or the CRPS that afflicts your life and your family's. What can you appreciate about your children feeling cheated and angry when pain limits your participation in their lives? Maybe your spouse has tired of the restrictions your pain puts on your relationship, your family, and possibly your financial stability. How can you possibly be grateful for those difficult issues? Being grateful is not about pain or other problems; it is about concentrating on the positives in life. It's easy to lose sight of this concept when you feel that you are a prisoner of pain. But even on your most painful day, there are many things to appreciate. It may take a bit of effort at first, but focusing on the good in your life and what you have, rather than what you do not have, heightens your appreciation for the world you live in rather than negating it.

If you feel that you have nothing to be grateful for, look around and think again about what you take for granted. Your mind might jump directly to your car, home, or other material possessions. Are you thankful for your favorite pair of jeans, that TV show you hate to miss, or the anchovy pizza that can be at your door just 20 minutes after you order it? How about all the positives in your life: your five senses, your family and friends, past memories and future hopes, your children's laughter? Surely you are grateful for your son's (or grandson's) crayon drawing stuck to the refrigerator door, or your daughter's sunny disposition. Nothing is too small or insignificant. Put pen to paper (or fingers to keyboard) and see if you don't run out of space before you run out of ideas for your gratitude list. If nothing comes to mind, confine your thoughts to a particular room in the house, a specific place or individual.

Count your blessings. Cultivate an attitude of gratitude. Some people maintain a daily gratitude journal, beginning or ending each day by jotting down three or four things (or an entire page) for which they are grateful. (Research indicates that gratitude journaling also enhances sleep.)[11] Give yourself a strong daily dose of gratitude to help deal with your pain. Do it every day and you will discover something miraculous. You will feel much better. You will also shift your energy to a more positive point of view that will attract more of what you want in life. You might feel that you have less to appreciate in life than others have, and some days may seem to hold little for which you can be thankful, but you need not let your pain interfere with the goodness and the positive aspects of your life.

THE POWER OF A GRATEFUL PERSPECTIVE

ANNA'S LIFE ABRUPTLY CHANGED when a bus slammed into her as she crossed a busy street. The accident left her with an injured back, broken ribs, and the loss of her left leg. When she came to us three months later, her back and ribs were healing, but the phantom leg pain was not. We designed a multidisciplinary treatment program that included psychotherapy, physical therapy (including mirror box therapy), and neuropathic pain medications. All of these treatments contributed to Anna's recovery and helped to manage her residual pain, but her best pain-fighting tool was her incredibly positive outlook and grateful perspective. Anna viewed the loss of her leg and the pain she felt as hurdles that she could and would overcome. And although her recovery was anything but easy, she remained confident about her future, refusing to dwell on her misfortune. In spite of the obstacles facing her, Anna constantly expressed thanks for surviving her ordeal and appreciation for our treatment efforts. She worked hard to get better, celebrating every small improvement she made. She never allowed herself to become disappointed when her response to treatment was slow or when setbacks occurred. She refused to be bitter or dwell on her misfortune, focusing instead on getting her life back on track. Just nine months after the accident, Anna was back at work as a university law professor. She continued to have some pain, but she did not allow it to control her life. ☼

7. Giving

It is more blessed to give than to receive—it is also easy and requires no special training. Gratitude begets giving. The more you appreciate things in your life, the more you will want to give back by helping others. All religions preach the virtues of giving or service—acts that benefit someone else. To Christians, it is charitable work. Jews call monetary giving tzedakah and refer to helping others as chesed, or righteous acts. Muslims are obliged to tithe to the poor and Hindus are encouraged to perform seva (service). Serving the greater good is one antidote to an isolated, painful life. People in pain who routinely give to charity or perform other altruistic acts are healthier and happier. They are among the best-adjusted pain patients. When you concentrate on "How can I help?" you are less likely to focus on what is wrong with you or what you do not have (a day without pain). Giving expands our perspective beyond our individual selves. It enhances our spiritual growth, helping us to connect to the divine. The possibilities for giving are endless, and the effort you expend helping others will reap immeasurable returns.

. . . .

I was piloting a small airplane when the engine failed and I was forced to crash land. As a result, I incurred some injuries, the most serious of which was thought to be a fracture of my T-12 vertebra. After neurosurgery and many weeks of hospitalization and physical therapy, I regained full functionality, but despite medication, I have constant pain in my lower back, buttocks, and upper legs. Working with a pain-management clinic, I had a neurostimulator and a pain pump implanted. The stimulator does not completely block my neuropathic pain, but it does provide relief for an hour or two, and it is helpful when I try to sleep. The pump supplies constant medication directly to my spinal column. I am able to supplement the dose, but I rarely need to do so. I still take some oral pain medication, but the pump provides the most effective pain relief without requiring that the drugs first pass through my organs. I do not know how I could tolerate my pain without it.

For me there are also mental elements dealing with my pain. The first is a determination to continue the normal activities of my life, which are already reduced due to age. I am aided by a caring wife who constantly motivates me to do the best I can. I am also inspired by my son, who suffered from a rare bone disease and spent much of his young life in body casts. Finally, there is the spiritual element, which is hard to define or describe. Primary is the belief that life must be lived. In addition, I believe that an element of sacrifice is sometimes expected. This can be in service to others, but also in an acceptance of life's circumstances. I find this spiritual element through faith in my religion. Others may find it elsewhere.

—Fred

Finding Help for Spiritual Growth

If you need help with the idea of spiritual strength as a means to cope with pain, many nonjudgmental resources await. Confer with your priest, minister, or rabbi, or ask your doctor to suggest a resource to help you work through spiritual issues. As health care professionals develop a growing recognition of their patients' comprehensive needs, spiritual resources are becoming easier to find. Many institutions offer spiritual meditation classes and have chaplains who are trained to provide interdenominational counseling.

SUMMARY POINTS
- **We are spiritual beings.**
- **Spiritual health positively impacts chronic pain.**
- **You may not be able to eliminate your pain, but you can limit its impact on your life.**
- **Prayer, meditation, gratitude, and service can help you cope with pain.**

The Family in Pain

Family dynamics are often complex, and a family's balance and harmony amid individual personalities and priorities can be tenuous at best. Adding chronic pain into the mix can be a disruptive or devastating influence that shifts the operating rhythm of the most closely knit households.

Chronic pain forces you to give up certain things, make allowances, and accept new limits. It imposes restrictions that change your world, and it can affect your family in the same way. The more pain keeps you from being your normal self, the greater the danger of upending the household's established, comfortable routine. You may argue more with your partner and children and become less involved in their lives. As you struggle with your pain, tension may build and tempers may flare as family members develop their own dysfunctional symptoms (table 8.1). This more likely occurs when pain becomes the family's new focus and seems to overshadow all else. Like you, family members may feel a loss of control because they cannot make your pain go away or return the household to its previous painless environment. Partners, children, and elderly parents living in the home may not accept this new normal or may be resentful of extra responsibilities that leave them little time for other activities and interests.

Families that do not ordinarily engage in open, honest discussion will have a particularly difficult time. Individuals may be reluctant to voice their opinions about the situation, and with no outlet to express themselves, they may stifle their feelings and become withdrawn or depressed or develop other worrisome issues. If the situation continues without

TABLE 8.1 Unhealthy emotions in a family with chronic pain

Emotion	Felt by the person in pain	Felt by the partner or spouse	Felt by other family members
Guilt	Because I am a burden to my family; my reduced contributions to the family require sacrifices by others.	Because I feel trapped by my partner's pain.	Because I cannot help enough or fix the problem; because I do not share my loved one's pain. Children: My parent's pain is my fault.
Fear	That I will never get better.	That my hopes and dreams will never be fulfilled.	That the family will never be the same.
Anger or resentment	Because my life is ruined; because I don't deserve this pain.	Because I have no cure; because the health insurance may not cover payments; because I have extra responsibilities; because my partner does not try hard enough or uses pain as a crutch.	Because the person in pain is not getting better; because of missed social, professional, and recreational activities.
Loss	Of independence, self-identity, and the way life used to be.	Of shared emotional and physical intimacy and financial security; it feels as if I've lost my partner.	Of relationships within the family as they used to be.
Sadness	For what life has become; that pain isolates me physically and emotionally.	That the future will not be as we had hoped.	For our disrupted lives.

resolution, relatives may become emotionally disconnected from one another, perpetuating dysfunction in a household where everyone is stuck in a rut of unhappiness.

Impact of Pain on Your Spouse or Partner

The stress and strain of seeing you struggle with life-altering pain can be difficult for your spouse or partner. Chronic pain can certainly test the bond between two people. Many couples find it to be a hardship that strengthens the closeness and trust they share. But one individual's pain can also weaken a relationship, particularly one that is already fragile. Emotional distance can develop when your partner shows no empathy for your plight, believes that your pain is not real, or suspects that you exaggerate its intensity or frequency. Sometimes people do not understand why their mates cannot just "snap out" of their pain or "work through" it. Individuals who feel this way are more likely to respond with anger rather than support. Partners frequently feel threatened by issues they cannot control or fix. Not knowing how to cope with your pain, your partner may simply ignore the situation, a response that might seem uncaring to you. You may then feel sad or bitter that you are not getting the understanding and support you need and deserve.

Communication is critical in all relationships, particularly those that are already strained. Talking about these problems can be uncomfortable, but avoiding discussion of pain and the problems it creates only makes a bad predicament worse. Even in the best of situations, frustrations can mount when painful flareups occur—the path of pain management is sometimes littered with setbacks, and even the smallest roadblock may seem enormous.

Unquestionably, your spouse's response to painful behavior affects your physical and emotional health. Research tells us that women are more likely to express their pain, while men tend to hide theirs—these are behaviors that our culture reinforces. Surprisingly, a study involving 78 couples with one spouse who had chronic fibromyalgia, osteoarthritis, or back pain contradicts previous research showing that women experience more pain, anxiety, and depression. In this study, men with chronic pain were more sensitive to their partner's responses and were more likely to respond negatively when their spouses were less respectful or accepting of their pain.[1] The study authors suggested that pain might be more disruptive to a man's traditional roles, creating more feelings of vulnerability and emotional upheaval when he does not receive support from his partner. Another study of 106 couples found that people catastrophize their pain more and experience greater disability when spousal support does not meet their expectations.[2]

Partners of people with chronic pain face difficult challenges of their own. When an individual loses functionality and mobility, the spouse often takes on more household and parental duties, even when the person in pain may only want him to listen to her concerns and support her emotionally, not necessarily do more around the house. Taking on unfamiliar or less traditional responsibilities may create feelings of irritation or bitterness. Financial concerns, the most common cause of divorce, can develop if you are unable to work, or if your partner must work longer hours to make up for declining income. In some families, partners need to reduce their work hours to care for the person in pain, further reducing family income and increasing the fiscal burdens. These matters might cause you to feel that you are a poor provider or that you are not carrying your share of the family's financial load.

Intimacy is often the first casualty in a relationship that is overshadowed by one person's pain. Stress can quickly deplete sexual interest and energy, and intercourse may be too painful. The nature of the relationship between two people may also change, so that their roles shift to patient and caretaker rather than husband and wife or domestic partners. Depending on the severity of an individual's chronic pain, intimacy need not be forsaken, but it might call for more spontaneity (whenever you feel up to it), less spontaneity (planning around times when your medication kicks in or when you usually have less pain), or a bit of creativity. In any case, it is one of those subjects that benefits from heart-to-heart discussion.

Impact of Pain on the Children

It is natural to want to shield your children from stressful topics or assume they are too young to understand, but kids usually pick up on tension in the family. They know when a parent is upset, even when they do not understand why. Seeing you in pain can be a scary situation for your children. They may become worried and afraid if they are confused about what is going on. Your own irritability or mood swings can cause them to react with guilt or temper tantrums. They may be disappointed about your reduced involvement in their lives, and little ones probably will not understand if you can no longer hold them or give them piggyback rides.

Children are sensitive to modifications in routine. So when something changes, it is always better to explain rather than ignore the situation. For younger children, saying that "Mommy has a headache," or "Dad's medicine makes him tired" may be all that is necessary. Older children can handle more complexity and may want more details. Your kids will benefit from understanding that some days are better than others for you and that even if you are sometimes out of sorts or cranky because you do not feel well, they are not to blame. Your pain can be an opportunity to teach them about stress and how to cope with it. The challenge is to tend to your own stress level while also protecting your child's well-being.

Tips for talking with children about pain:

- Use simple, age-appropriate terms to describe your condition or your actions.

- Realize that all children process issues differently. Try to honor your child's wishes; provide as little or as much information as he wants to know.
- Encourage your children to talk about their feelings and ask questions.
- Listen closely and honestly address their concerns.
- Reassure them that your pain is not their fault and that you love them even when you have pain.
- Create alternative ways of comforting your children if you cannot pick them up or hug them.
- Keep the lines of communication open, especially if your children develop bad behavior.
- Keep their lives as normal as possible.

Behaviors That Reinforce Pain and Sabotage Recovery

Watching someone you love wage daily war against pain can be heartbreaking. Family support can help the person cope, but for various reasons, loved ones do not always react in supportive ways. In some instances, pain forges convoluted relationships. It is only natural to want to help someone who is in pain, especially someone we care about. But being overly protective or too solicitous does a disservice to the person in pain. The line between providing too much support and not enough is thin. As harsh as it may sound, over-sympathizing reinforces helplessness; actions fueled by pity, sorrow, or guilt are not the best way to bolster someone you love. Acting on someone's behalf when she can act herself limits her opportunity to maintain her self-reliance (even though it may be limited) and sense of self-worth. It may also create an unhealthy codependency between the two of you. Automatically telling a spouse in pain, "Don't worry, I'll take care of that," regardless of his ability or desire to do things for himself, can foster more pain. Whether or not either partner realizes it, getting too much attention because of pain can become a reward that subconsciously reinforces the need for attention.

Another way families might unintentionally make a poor situation worse is by inadvertently encouraging inappropriate or bad behavior by the person in pain. When people in pain express their frustration and anger in hurtful ways, a little extra understanding and compassion can be just what the doctor ordered. Frequently, however, believing that someone in pain cannot help himself can give that person free rein to behave badly. A partner in pain may also "act out" more to prove that his pain is real or to get the support he needs. Another harmful element is the "secondary gains" people often experience from being sick or disabled: sympathy, increased attention, and release from responsibility. Although most people would gladly trade these "benefits" to be pain-free, some will welcome being exempt from work and chores, thrive on increased attention, and like having carte blanche for continually poor temper and unreasonable conduct. Problems develop when these benefits begin to outweigh the reduced activity, decreased social interaction, and other losses experienced because of pain. When this happens, the motivation to reduce pain becomes diminished, but a person rarely comes to this conclusion consciously. Such behavior is almost always subconscious. It is a hurdle that an experienced psychotherapist can help patients and families surmount.

An Action Plan for Family Harmony

You are not powerless in confronting the influence pain has on your family. There are many things you can do to preserve the bonds you share and make life easier for all of you.

- Talk about it. Honest and nonjudgmental communication between family members is essential to prevent pain from interfering in relationships. People who suffer with pain may be unaware of the stress they cause others in the family. Acknowledging these issues, as uncomfortable as that may be, and resolving to change behaviors is the only way to rescue the situation to everyone's satisfaction. Let your loved ones know how you feel. Your silence and emotional withdrawal may encourage their estrangement from you. When communication with your partner is strained, talking with a trusted friend or a member of the clergy who will listen and give you honest feedback can be helpful.

- Educate the family. Your family will not intuitively know what you are going through unless they have experienced chronic pain firsthand. It is difficult to accept all the ways pain changes lives, and relatives are usually less critical when they understand the nuances of a chronic condition. A meaningful pain-management strategy can then become a family concern: what helps the patient also leads to a brighter, less traumatic future for others.

- Consider counseling. When communication is difficult, a qualified therapist can help individuals, couples, and families navigate these complex concerns. Therapy provides a nonthreatening environment that facilitates healthy dialogue without fear of repercussion. It also helps families identify negative codependent behaviors and develop positive communication and coping skills. Family counseling sessions can be invaluable for educating individuals about chronic pain and helping them understand why a loved one feels and acts the way she does. Therapy can also help family members learn how to be caring without causing harm. Attending one-on-one therapy may also provide opportunities for family members to voice the sense of loss they feel and deal with related issues.

- Do what you can. Managing your normal tasks and responsibilities as much as possible will reduce the extra responsibilities your family members need to take on. Pace yourself. Instead of automatically saying no to family activities and tasks, try replacing those you can no longer perform with those you can, so that you maintain an active and contributing role in the family—this can boost your feelings of self-worth.

- Stay connected. Persistent pain increases the sense of isolation you feel when it cuts you off from the people you love. Make a point each day to interact with family, no matter how small the effort. A touch, a smile, or a short conversation can maintain the emotional connection we all need. The same holds true for friendships. Social withdrawal can have profoundly negative effects on your life and your family's life. A text, an e-mail, a social media posting, or a brief phone call can help you remain connected to and involved with people who are important in your life.

- Ask for help. Do not suffer in silence. Ask for assistance when you need it. Friends and family are often willing to help but may not know what they can and should do. Fear that they might offend you or make you feel less capable may make them reluctant to offer. Take the initiative to let the people who care about you know how they can help you.

- Accept what is. In a sense, living well with chronic pain requires all family members to accept that pain may always be a part of their lives but that life can go on. Families become closer and fare better when they understand that working to improve a painful condition is more rewarding than simply wishing for a magic cure.

☀ A FAMILY AFFLICTED WITH COMPLEX REGIONAL PAIN SYNDROME

SANDY WAS A HAPPY WIFE AND A BUSY MOTHER with two small daughters, a teenage son, and chronic regional pain syndrome. After several months of moderate symptoms, her muscle and joint pain escalated until it was constant and overwhelming. Sandy was always focused on her pain; she could not seem to redirect her thoughts toward much else. Caring for herself became difficult. She was miserable during the day and sleepless at night. After several doctors and numerous medications, Sandy's hope of returning to a normal life was fading. Exhausted from fighting pain all day and bitter that her life was not different, she spent much of her time in bed. She felt less motivated about treatment and became less involved with the life of her family. As her pain continued to erode her own happiness, it had devastating effects on her loved ones. With her husband working two jobs to pay the mounting medical bills, the bulk of household duties and parenting responsibilities for the girls fell to her son Dan—it was a burdensome role that quickly took its toll. Dan's sunny nature and enthusiasm gave way to uncharacteristic brooding and resentment. His once exceptional school grades plummeted.

By the time Sandy came to us, she had abandoned her prescribed medications and was taking handfuls of over-the-counter NSAIDs that irritated her stomach and failed to control her pain. We outlined a multifaceted regimen to manage Sandy's pain, lift her mood, and restore some semblance of her functionality. We replaced her NSAIDs with a low dose of a long-lasting opioid that kept a consistent level of analgesic in her system. We twice supplemented this with corticosteroid injections into her hips, a particularly troublesome source of pain. Although Sandy was initially skeptical of her ability to get up, get dressed, and move around, we encouraged her to attend twice-weekly physical conditioning sessions with a physical therapist experienced with CRPS. She began with minimal stretching while seated, slowly progressing to gentle movements that improved her range of motion and flexibility. Her pain therapy also included psychological counseling. Combined with an antidepressant, these sessions gave her new perspective and supplied her with coping tools to view her pain less negatively. With newly learned biofeedback techniques, Sandy gradually gained control over the anxiety that often triggered her painful symptoms. Weekly support group meetings with other people who had CRPS and who understood what she was going through also helped, and they lessened Sandy's feelings of isolation. Her psychotherapist recommended family counseling as well. Her husband refused to attend, so the situation was not ideal, but Dan did attend separate sessions with and without his mother, which encouraged more honest communication.

Sandy's progress made several starts and stops, but in time, the collective therapies resulted in positive change. She concentrated on living one day at a time, appreciating intervals when she had less pain and could do more. At her therapist's suggestion, she focused on three daily priorities: spending time with her family, engaging in some activity that she enjoyed, and performing at least one task that gave her a sense of accomplishment. She continued to experience symptoms, but in time Sandy functioned better on most days and was better able to care for herself and the girls, restoring a measure of her son's independence. ○

SUMMARY POINTS
- Chronic pain affects the entire family.
- The stress of dealing with persistent pain can strengthen or weaken family bonds.
- Discuss your condition in age-appropriate terms with your children.
- Communication and acceptance are the keys to surviving chronic pain with healthy family relationships intact.

9

The Patient in Control

People who live with pain often say that one of its worst aspects is the loss of control it creates, that losing the ability to live their lives normally slowly breaks them down until they feel and act like someone they are not.

Facing Your Fears

Pain is scary. The thought that it may continue to narrow your focus, limit your interactions, and constrain the quality of your life can be even more terrifying. You may fear that even the smallest movement will cause more debilitating pain and that your future holds more of the same. Perhaps you are afraid that the relief your medication provides will be only temporary, that sooner or later your intense pain will return. All these trepidations take their toll, perhaps making you feel that your life is in free fall without a safety net.

Although fear is a natural response to pain, it can trap you as effectively as a gorilla sitting on your chest. Living in angst suppresses motivation, paralyzing the inclination to get up, move around, think positively, and pursue the very therapies that will improve your condition and make your life better. Left untreated, fear invites unhappiness. It may grow until it becomes your primary focus: you may be apprehensive that you will get worse, doubt that your life will ever again be fulfilling, or be skeptical that you will ever be able to do the things you want to do. These feelings tend to make you overly cautious about what you do and how you move, so that you use your body less and it weakens, creating more pain and increasing your level of disability. Your own cultural convictions or beliefs may also hinder your ability to improve. You may avoid seeing a physician if you believe that toughing through pain is a sign of strength or that taking medication is only for the weak. You might feel guilty for complaining, or you may avoid treatment if you believe you would be wasting a physician's time. Perhaps you consider pain to be your lot in life, that nothing can be done to improve your condition. These fears are not uncommon, but they can increase your pain and add to your misery.

Because pain affects both body and mind, a single medication or therapy is unlikely to address all the physical and emotional problems pain creates. Following the right multidisciplinary management strategy will help you manage your misgivings, close pain gates (or at least move them in the right direction), and provide some measure of relief so that you become more independent from your pain. The right mixture of medications combined with the physical and emotional therapies described in previous chapters can help you defeat anxiety and keep a positive outlook for the present and the future. A qualified therapist can help you deal with these complicated issues.

Solving the Chronic Pain Puzzle

The path to relief begins with the question, "What is wrong with me?" but diagnosing chronic pain is easier said than done. A single visit to the doctor will probably not remedy your problem, because the underlying source of chronic pain, unlike acute pain, is often a Herculean riddle that refuses to be solved. Even when the source of pain is identified, a cure might not be possible, but in almost all cases, the pain can be reduced and the person's quality of life can be greatly improved.

Who should treat you? Pain is the most common reason for seeing a doctor and taking medication, yet doctors have no established standards for addressing chronic pain; that is why treatment strategies vary widely. You and your doctor (along with your entire health care team) are partners against pain. Your common goal should extend beyond simply treating symptoms. It should be to develop, and adjust as needed, a comprehensive treatment approach to accomplish the following objectives:

- reduce your pain and suffering
- decrease your anxiety, depression, fear, and frustration
- help you to sleep undisturbed by pain
- increase your self-confidence
- recover your ability to care for yourself and your family
- restore your ability to return to work, even though it may not be the same type of work you previously performed

Finding the Right Physician

The first step on the path to improvement is finding a physician who understands the nuances of pain. Treating chronic pain is a distinct medical specialty, and most physicians are not trained or experienced to deal with the complexities involved. Seeking relief can be a frustrating odyssey of doctor-hopping, taking overlapping medications with side effects that create new problems, and finding that after all is said and done, the pain remains.

If your relationship with your physician does not work well—if recommended therapies do not produce satisfactory results in a reasonable amount of time, or if your pain becomes worse—it is time to seek a second opinion. Ask your primary physician for a referral to a pain specialist or a pain clinic that offers multiple therapies under a single roof. Or use the "Find a Physician" tool on the website of the American Academy of Pain Medicine (www.painmed.org). Ideally, you want a doctor whose practice is devoted to treating chronic pain. A pain specialist may be the principal treating physician who provides treatment and coordinates other aspects of your care with other health care professionals. Some specialists treat most types of chronic pain; others specialize in specific conditions. Your physician should be a person whom you would describe this way:

- expresses concern about how pain affects your life
- takes you seriously

- listens compassionately as you describe your symptoms
- inspires your confidence and trust
- understands the wide range of pain medications and other treatment options
- explains what you can realistically expect from treatment
- considers alternatives when treatment fails or causes intolerable side effects
- works with you to understand your pain and treat it

Your physician uses a variety of tools to assess your symptoms, determine what is causing the pain, and rule out what is not. These essential steps may include the following:

- a full medical history
- your description of the pain
- a thorough examination
- blood tests and other lab work
- x-rays, CT or MRI scans, or other diagnostics

✻ RELIEF AFTER THE RIGHT DIAGNOSIS

TOM, A RETIRED PARK RANGER IN HIS EARLY EIGHTIES, suffered with a painful back and a burning sensation in his right foot. He assumed it would get better on its own, but when it continued for three years without relief, he finally decided a visit to his doctor was in order. After a variety of tests, his doctor diagnosed sciatica with referred pain into the foot. He gave Tom a prescription for hydrocodone and a sheet of recommended back exercises to be performed every day. This diagnosis made perfect sense to Tom, because the symptoms, as described by his physician and according to what Tom read on the Internet, seemed to match his pain. Having lived with the affliction for so long, Tom was happy to have a diagnosis, and he looked forward to getting back to walking, gardening, and other activities that he had given up because they aggravated his condition. But after two weeks of taking the medication and performing the exercises, he had no noticeable improvement. He returned to his physician, who suggested that Tom give the regimen a bit more time. Several weeks later, when

Tom was still no better, his physician referred him to a physical therapist for biweekly stretching exercises.

After four more weeks he was no better, and in fact, Tom's symptoms were worse. He was frustrated and depressed, thinking that nothing would help him and his condition might never improve. At that point, his doctor suggested a spinal cord stimulator as a last resort. Although Tom was not completely comfortable with the idea of surgery, he agreed and proceeded with the operation to install the device. That treatment also failed. Tom was then referred to our pain clinic. We conducted a full physical workup, and when we closely questioned him about the nature of his symptoms, we learned that Tom's minor sciatica was not his most serious problem. While it was annoying, it was tolerable and did not curtail his activities or lifestyle. His foot pain was more severe. He could barely touch his foot to the ground without pain. We determined that the primary source of pain was not his spine but arthritis and bone spurs in his foot. We directed his physical therapist to focus on his foot, and gradually, Tom regained nearly normal functionality and mobility. ○

Making the Most of Physician Appointments

With a bit of preparation, you can make sure that you get your questions answered and make the most of the limited time you have with your physician.

Be prepared. When you schedule an initial appointment with a physician, ask what records or other information you should bring with you. Keep a pain log documenting the intensity, severity, and frequency of your pain and what you were doing just before it occurred; this record will help you identify pain triggers and nonobvious pain patterns. Bring a list of all of the prescribed and over-the-counter medications, supplements, and herbs you take and the results of your most recent diagnostic tests or scans. Be prepared to discuss your family's medical history, so that your physician can determine whether your pain might be related to a hereditary syndrome (table 9.1).

Do your homework. An informed patient is an empowered patient. Learn as much as you can about your condition and symptoms before

TABLE 9.1   Patient tools

Tool	Purpose
Medication and allergy list	Identifies substances that cause an allergic reaction and informs the doctor of all the medications you take
Pain log	Helps to monitor the details of your pain
Interactive pain map	Shows the locations of your pain and tracks your progress over time
Daily activity list	Records your level of functionality from day to day
Preappointment summary	Summarizes essential information for your appointment
After-appointment follow-up card	Helps you keep track of your doctor's recommendations

Note: The website of the American Chronic Pain Association (www.theACPA.org) includes these easy-to-use patient tools.

your appointment, so that you can discuss them with your physician. The more you understand your condition, the better off you will be.

Prioritize your issues. Before each appointment, think about what you would like to accomplish during your brief time with the physician: discuss a medication's undesirable side effects, understand more about your treatment alternatives, or ask for a referral. You probably won't have time to ask all your questions, so plan ahead to ask the right ones. Prioritize and write down the two or three issues for which you most need your doctor's input.

Bring someone with you. Studies show that patients forget about half of what they hear during a doctor's visit. That's not surprising, especially for someone who is dealing with intense pain. Four ears are always better than two. If you can, bring someone else with you to take notes. Or record your conversation so you can replay it later at home.

Speak up. The most beneficial consultations are interactive. Try not to be shy about your pain. Ask, if you need a particular treatment or a bewildering term explained or repeated. Suggest that your physician draw a diagram or use plain language to define a term or clarify a procedure. Honest communication with your physician is essential. Express your fears, doubts, or confusion, and say what is on your mind. Tell your doctor how you truly feel or what you want to know, rather than what you think he wants to hear. Ideally, you will leave your doctor's appointment with a sense of clarity about your diagnosis, treatment options, and the prescribed path forward. Understand how to take your medication, what effects you can expect (and how to deal with them), when you might begin to feel relief, and what other therapies you should begin.

Be ready to describe your pain. Pain is subjective, and people have different amounts of tolerance for it. One person's level 4 might be another's level 8. Doctors have no other way to measure or understand it than the description you provide. How does it feel? Describing your pain as succinctly as possible will help your physician diagnose the cause. Is it dull or sharp? Is it stabbing, throbbing, aching, burning, tingling, gnawing, stinging, pounding, pulsing, shooting, radiating, searing, tearing, pinching, splitting, or crushing? An honest and accurate explanation of your pain characteristics will help your physician diagnose the underlying cause and recommend appropriate treatment (table 9.2).

Reconfirm what you hear. Before you leave the office, restate what you think you heard, to make sure your understanding is correct. Summarize conclusions and next steps: for example, you will start a particular medication immediately, and you will begin physical therapy two weeks before returning for your next appointment. Ask about articles, books, DVDs, and any other educational information your doctor recommends to increase your knowledge and understanding.

Living Well with Pain

No one who lives in pain wants to stay that way. But it is not always easy to make meaningful behavioral changes in life, even when they can move you toward what you want. Inertia, whether it is emotional or physical, is a powerful force. It is the path of least resistance when pain and other barriers in life keep us from being happy or healthy, and it can be the most difficult to overcome. Your motivation to live your best life is what defines the difference between a painful existence and a rewarding life despite pain.

Living better with chronic pain means establishing a new normal. It is an ongoing learning experience that requires you to accept that pain

TABLE 9.2 Describing your pain

Questions	Details
When did it start?	After an injury healed, following surgery, or out of the blue?
Where is it?	If you can, show your doctor exactly where you feel the pain.
When does it occur?	Is it constant or worse during certain times of the day or night?
Does it affect more than one area of your body?	Is it localized on one side of your head? Does it begin in the back and travel down one leg?
How long does it last?	Does it recede or disappear at certain times of the day or night, or is it always with you?
How does it feel?	What sensations do you feel?
How intense or severe is it?	Is it more of a "slows-you-down-but-you-can-still-function" or an "I-just-cannot-take-it" kind of pain? Rate your pain on a scale from 0 to 10, with 0 being no pain (perhaps between episodes) and 10 being the worst pain imaginable.
What treatments have you tried?	What worked and what did not?
What makes it worse?	Does your pain increase with certain food triggers, specific movements, or positions?
What makes it better?	Does cold, heat, or massage reduce the level or intensity? Does physical therapy help?

forces you to give up certain things and discover alternative ways to accomplish others. You might replace running with biking, swimming, or walking. Try tai chi or yoga instead of more strenuous workouts. If you can no longer perform your previous full-time job, perhaps you can work part-time or transition to a less painful position or occupation. The same philosophy applies to personal interactions. You might need to prioritize and limit activities with the family or settle for coffee or dinner with friends instead of the bustling social life or frequent entertaining you enjoyed previously.

Realize that the road to pain control can be long and frustrating, especially when new medications or treatments do not live up to your expectations. Ideally, your first visit to a physician will bring you the relief you seek. More often, successful pain management is a trial-and-error process. The clearest path to a fuller, more satisfying life requires fortitude and patience to determine what combination of therapies gives you the best results. Do not give up! For most people, improvement occurs gradually, and sometimes the reprieve from pain is short-lived. Your physician and your extended health care team will help guide you toward the best possible decisions. You, however, are in the driver's seat. More than anyone else, you know what makes you feel better or worse, and you control what you do about your pain.

Living a Better Life

You need not concede your life to pain. You can get better. It will not happen until you make pain management your priority—you need a sense of mission about this. Your actions and thoughts are most critical to achieving a better outlook and a better life. You can do much to manage your care, your body, your mind, and the logistics of living so that you live a full and enjoyable life. Use all the tools at your disposal (figure 9.1) to minimize your pain as much as possible and move beyond it so that it becomes something that you manage and live with and does not become who you are. Take one day at a time, building forward momentum toward improvement. Set realistic, achievable, short-term goals, such as exercising for a few more minutes each day to gradually improve your stamina and endurance. Take time to engage in activities that build physical and emotional strength. Stay motivated, so that you stick to your recovery plan even on days when you are physically and mentally exhausted and want to give up. Continue despite setbacks. Learn to control your pain and live without fear so that you can move on with your life. Gather your courage, maintain a positive attitude, and take responsibility for your own well-being. As much as possible, consider and plan for the future, rather than dwelling on the past.

You can extricate yourself from the control pain exerts on your life. It is not always easy, and improvement is not likely to occur overnight, particularly if your pain is severe, but it is possible. Chronic pain is a bump in the road that may not disappear, and it may be more formidable at some times, but you can find ways to go over it or around it.

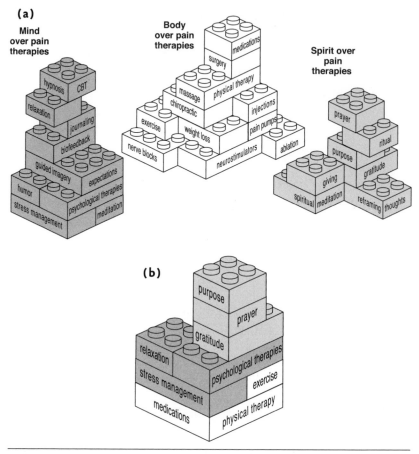

FIGURE 9.1. Numerous mind, body, and spiritual tools provide building blocks that help to reduce pain and rise above it (*a*). Layering individual therapies together (*b*) is the most effective method of living well with chronic pain.

. . . .

My journey with complex regional pain syndrome began in 2009 after two failed neuroma surgeries. The pain was constant, unrelenting. I kept thinking "Why me? I want my life back!" I lost my job and I was struggling to keep up with things in life I had previously taken for granted. Finding a doctor who knew anything about this disease, let alone believed it actually was one, was not easy. My research led me to a pain specialist who was encouraging, compassionate, and honest about the realities of treating CRPS. I felt confident that he could help me. As part of his approach to managing my pain, he encouraged me to consult with a pain psychologist. Once when we were discussing a par-

ticular treatment, the psychologist asked, "What happens if it doesn't work?" I thought the answer was obvious: I will keep on trying. Today, I am still a work in progress. I have learned to manage my pain with daily medications and guided imagery exercise, along with physical therapy twice a month and nerve blocks. It is not easy, and it did not happen overnight. With my family's love and support and my doctor's perseverance, the quality of my life has greatly improved. I am once again a wife and a mother, rather than the patient I have been for the last three years. While I don't accept my pain, I have learned to manage it and never give up or lose hope.

—Suzanne

SUPPORT GROUPS

Sometimes the comfort you need comes from others who know firsthand what you are going through. Sharing your feelings, whether face-to-face or virtually, decreases feelings of isolation and helps you relax. Many hospitals and pain clinics coordinate local support-group meetings, and the websites of the U.S. Pain Foundation (www.uspainfoundation.org) and the American Chronic Pain Association (www.theacpa.org) will help you find support groups in your area. To find online chronic pain forums, search for "chronic pain support group" or a specific type of pain, such as "fibromyalgia support group." Look for people who provide positive advice and support, rather than those who dwell on misery and the downsides of pain.

SUMMARY POINTS

- **Fear intensifies the pain experience and decreases the motivation to get better.**
- **Improvement usually occurs gradually, and finding the right combination of therapies may take time and include setbacks.**
- **You can get better when you make pain management your priority.**
- **Many tools are available to help you manage your pain and live well.**
- **Take control; don't allow the path of least resistance to be your guide.**

The Future of Pain Management

Chronic pain is a global problem of enormous proportion that needs and deserves far more attention than it currently receives. An aging population and soaring rates of obesity, diabetes, and other pain-related health issues are increasing the number of people affected and driving the demand for better solutions. We are no longer content to simply ask, "Where does it hurt?" and to treat all pain (or all individuals with pain) in the same way. Even more, "Just learn to live with it" is no longer a satisfactory medical response.

We are more knowledgeable about pain than we were even a decade ago. We understand more about pain pathways, stimuli that manipulate pain gates, and how the mind influences perception. These discoveries represent welcome progress, and our arsenal of tools continues to expand. Yet many questions remain unanswered, and we still have much to learn to enhance the value of pain care. Studying chronic pain is no small challenge, because its sources are many, they are complex, and they are influenced by so many diverse factors.

A Better System?

Today, a person in pain is disadvantaged because the splintered medical system does not always acknowledge or meet the person's needs. Most Americans are treated by general practitioners or primary physicians in managed-care plans. These doctors are used to treating common ail-ments with standard medications but have little or no training or expe-rience with pain management. Despite its many advantages and cost efficiencies, the managed-care infrastructure is not designed to support the extra time and effort doctors need to spend with pain patients or to provide the specialized care needs of the individual with chronic pain. A pain specialist is often considered only as a last resort, after ordinary treatments fail to make a meaningful difference in a patient's life. Even when a physician recognizes the need for a referral to a pain specialist, most patients, especially those who live outside metropolitan areas, do not have reasonable access to a pain doctor or a pain-management clinic. The implications are stunning: many people are forced to endure pain-fully limited lives because medications, nerve blocks, neural stimulators, pain pumps, or other advanced treatments are beyond their reach.

Although more physicians are becoming credentialed pain specialists, our health care system must shift to support more timely, better out-comes for people with pain. Since the primary physician is likely to re-main the core of individual medical care, training must be retooled to give new generations of treating physicians the skills they need to ade-quately assess and treat pain; this would also reduce the current prob-lems of underprescribing and overprescribing medications. All medical students need more than a cursory introduction to pain if we expect them to adequately address symptoms and recognize when the needs of their patients exceed their own capabilities. To that end, we must also foster collaborative relationships between treating physicians and pain specialists. Patient education is another area where significant improve-ment can be made.

Looking Forward

Five trends in the scientific and medical communities are poised to make changes that will benefit pain patients.

1. Enhanced Medications

Medication is likely to remain the primary treatment for most patients with intractable pain. While analgesics work well for certain types of pain, we need innovative medicinal approaches that produce results without troublesome side effects, particularly for neuropathic pain. At best, however, the process of introducing new medicine is slow and limited to two primary methods: either modify the use of existing drugs or engineer new formulations that work in different ways.

Progressive imaging technologies are broadening our view of how emotional and sensory centers of the brain process pain and react to different treatments. Eventually, this type of information will enable pharmaceutical companies to refine analgesic formulations so that they are faster-acting, more effective, and have fewer side effects. A good deal of laboratory work is now focusing on improving opioids. One such medicine is morphine-6-0 sulfate, a pain reliever that is more potent and longer-lasting than morphine but does not appear to cause constipation, a common side effect of opioids. Pharmaceutical researchers are also working to develop a potent morphine-like drug that relieves pain without sedating effects. Other efforts are under way to decrease tolerance to morphine-based medications and make opioids abuse-resistant.

Every improvement made to an existing medication is a step in the right direction, but realizing innovative advancement in pain treatment will require the development of new drugs that are engineered to work in different ways. Although the ideal pain drug may not be close on the horizon, expanding on recent discoveries may provide information that encourages pharmaceutical companies to develop new treatments. One promising area of emerging research is the manipulation of receptors to control pain. Current analgesics target only a limited number of pain receptors; identifying new receptors could provide new opportunities for next-generation pain medications. In 2012, American and Australian researchers announced that opioids activate an immune receptor in the brain, creating an inflammatory response that promotes opioid tolerance. Future opioids built on this knowledge could block this immune receptor, promoting morphine-based benefits without the tradeoff of undesirable side effects.[1]

Scientists are rethinking the potential of targeting kappa receptors as gate-closing mechanisms. Clinical trials during the 1980s were abandoned when agonist medications using these receptors were found to cause depression and hallucinations. More recent attention is directed to potential kappa agonists that do not enter the central nervous system and therefore do not unleash these unwanted effects. The notion of targeting different receptors is also bolstered by emerging research involving substance P. In laboratory tests with animals, a cocktail of substance P and the chemical saporin produced positive results. Within days of the injections, the concoction entered targeted receptors for substance P and the saporin destroyed the pain-transmitting neurons along the entire length of the spinal cord.[2]

Another area of study has to do with *ion channels,* pathways along cell membranes where electrically charged particles enter and exit cells. Barely researched until a few years ago, ion channels are involved extensively in nerve functions, including the transport of pain messages. Research of this type may result in new therapies for hard-to-treat neuropathic pain.

More effective methods of delivery are also likely. We can expect more medicines in the form of nasal sprays, inhalants, skin patches, and formulations that are pushed through the skin without a needle. These new deliveries will speed medication directly to areas of the brain that control and perceive pain, bypassing the intestinal tract and reducing gastrointestinal side effects.

The frontier of pain medicine for specific chronic conditions is also promising. Even though the causes of many conditions still elude us, research is testing creative approaches to fibromyalgia, chronic regional pain syndrome, and other conditions that cause widespread pain. Preliminary studies, for example, show that people with CRPS have antibodies that are created by their own autoimmune response and that immunotherapy with intravenous immunoglobulins served them better than conventional medications.[3] These findings expand our understanding of this devastating disease and may help us find new treatment strategies that focus on the immune system.

2. Genetic Discovery

Why do some people develop chronically painful conditions when others do not? And why do two persons with the same pain respond differently to the same treatment? Part of the answer in both cases is genetics. Consider rheumatoid arthritis, an autoimmune disease that develops when a genetic predisposition is triggered by environmental factors. Genetics determines the severity of an individual's RA symptoms and how the person's body metabolizes and responds to different treatments.

Dozens of genes that affect chronic pain have been identified, and many others will surely be discovered. The explosion of data regarding human genetics is driving improvements in all areas of medicine. Future genetic testing might help physicians choose treatments based on an individual's unique genetic profile, rather than our current approach of making one type of drug available and hoping that it works for many people. Ultimately, we hope that genetics and pharmacogenetics will reveal more about how the body processes painful stimuli, and specifically, how genes drive gender-specific differences in pain intensity and perception. This is the promise of personalized medicine: two people who have the same migraine headaches would be treated differently if screening tests show that one of them lacks a particular gene function or has a faulty receptor. In time, we may be able to read an individual's genetic signature to predict how she will respond to certain types of NSAIDs, opioids, or other analgesics, thus eliminating much of the trial-and-error process.

One of the most exciting medical frontiers is the harnessing of stem cells, the body's own blank slates, to repair damaged tissue or regenerate new muscle, bone, or tissue. Stem cell therapy is already used to replace bone marrow in leukemia patients, and one day it may be key to treatment for degenerative conditions. Veterinarians are already using stem cell therapy to treat arthritis in animals. If the same (or a similar) procedure proves to be safe and effective for humans, cell-based therapies might one day strike arthritis and other disorders from our list of incurable conditions. Testing new medications directly on stem cells, rather than animals, could speed the delivery of new medications. But producing viable stem cell treatments to rebuild or replace damaged nerves, bone, joints, or tissue may be years away.

3. Neurotransmitter Regulation and Replacement

We are just beginning to understand how extensively neurotransmitter deficiencies affect mental and physical health. People who lack adequate serotonin, for example, may develop mood and sleep disorders, and people who have insufficient dopamine may have inhibited signaling between nerves. (Parkinson's disease develops when nerves in the brain are no longer able to release dopamine.) Imbalance in the levels of certain neurotransmitters can also cause pain, as appears to be the case with fibromyalgia and chronic fatigue syndrome. Levels of adrenaline, serotonin, norepinephrine, histamine, and other neurotransmitters may be disturbed in individuals with these conditions.

In the future, the diagnosis of painful conditions might involve routine screenings to identify irregular levels of neurotransmitters, which could then be regulated with medications or with lifestyle and dietary changes. Some pharmaceutical companies are working to synthesize endorphins, norepinephrine, and other neurotransmitter-like chemicals that would mimic the body's natural painkillers.

4. Neurostimulation

As our knowledge about disrupting pain signals expands and our skill increases, neurostimulators will likely become more sophisticated. Already, newer "smart" stimulators automatically adjust the amount and location of electricity sent, based on a person's body movement.

Repetitive transcranial magnetic stimulation (rTMS) is a breakthrough treatment for anxiety disorders and depression that resist medication and psychotherapy. rTMS uses a large electromagnetic coil, which is placed against the patient's scalp near the forehead. The coil is pulsed on and off for 30 to 40 minutes, producing a mild tapping on the forehead as electrical currents move through the skull and excite brain neurons that regulate depression and mood. Unlike other brain-stimulation procedures, rTMS does not require surgery or anesthesia, so it can be performed as an outpatient procedure. The treatment is painless, although some patients experience temporary mild headaches, spasming facial muscles, or dizziness. Pain relief from rTMS is somewhat longer-lasting than stimulation with electrodes. Some researchers have found that repeated applications significantly reduce pain for people who suffer with chronic regional pain syndrome.[4] Other research has shown that rTMS can relieve pain, at least temporarily, for individuals with fibromyalgia or neuropathic pain.[5] So far, studies of rTMS are promising, but additional research is needed to determine whether it is a viable method of long-term pain control and to learn which neural sites are most advantageous for stimulation.

5. Increased Integration of Multidisciplinary Therapies

Medicine will probably always be an integral part of pain treatment, but it is not the only treatment or the most effective means of managing pain for all people. While the medical community as a whole does not entirely support the idea of integrative medicine, more health care professionals and patients alike embrace the importance of a comprehensive approach that treats the whole patient rather than singular symptoms. Evidence-based studies and education are keys to recognizing that the most effective prescription for chronic pain is a combination of medication, physical therapy, psychotherapy, and self-management. Standards for treating chronic pain—which have not yet been developed—need to emphasize holistic treatment that addresses a patient's physical, emotional, psychological, and spiritual well-being.

Will Pain Become a Problem of the Past?

Eliminating chronic pain is a tall order; it may well be impossible. But if we can successfully overcome the social, economic, and political hurdles that stand in our way, scientific discovery will provide answers that will soften the harsh edges of lives marred by pain. It is just a matter of time.

Notes

Introduction

1. *Relieving Pain in America: A Blueprint for Transforming Prevention, Care, Education, and Research*. Institute of Medicine, June 2011.

2. Blumenthal D, Gokhale M, Campbell EG, et al. "Preparedness for clinical practice: Reports of graduating residents at academic health centers." *Journal of the American Medical Association* 286, no. 9 (2001): 1027-34.

Chapter 1. The Science of Pain

1. Baliki MN, Geha PY, Apkarian AV, et al. "Beyond feeling: Chronic pain hurts the brain, disrupting the default-mode network dynamics." *Journal of Neuroscience* 28, no. 6 (2008): 1398-1403.

2. Sakai K, Matsuno H, Tsuji H, et al. "Substance P receptor (NK1) gene expression in synovial tissue in rheumatoid arthritis and osteoarthritis." *Scandinavian Journal of Rheumatology* 27, no. 2 (1998): 135-41; Anichini M, Cesaretti S, Lepori M, et al. "Substance P in the serum of patients with rheumatoid arthritis." *Revue du Rhumatisme* (English edition) 64, no. 1 (1997): 18-21; "Russell IJ, Orr MD, Littman B, et al. "Elevated cerebrospinal fluid levels of substance P in patients with the fibromyalgia syndrome." *Arthritis and Rheumatism* 37, no. 11 (1994): 1593-1601.

3. Levine JD, Gordon NC, Fields HL. "The mechanism of placebo analgesia." *Lancet* 2, no. 8091 (1978): 654-57.

4. Guo JY, Wang JY, Luo F. "Dissection of placebo analgesia in mice: The conditions for activation of opioid and non-opioid systems." *Journal of Psychopharmacology* 24, no. 10 (2010): 1561-67.

5. Kaptchuk TJ, Friedlander E, Kelley JM, et al. "Placebos without deception: A randomized controlled trial in irritable bowel syndrome." *PLoS ONE* 5, no. 12 (2010): e15591.

6. Leresche L. "Defining gender disparities in pain management." *Clinical Orthopaedics and Related Research* 469, no. 7 (2011): 1871-77; Hoffmann DE, Tarzian AJ. "The girl who cried pain: A bias against women in the treatment of pain." *Journal of Law, Medicine, and Ethics* 28, no. s4 (2001): 13-27.

7. Ruau D, Liu LY, Clark JD, et al. "Sex differences in reported pain across 11,000 patients captured in electronic medical records." *Journal of Pain* 13, no. 3 (2012): 228-34; Mowlavi A, Cooney D, Febus L, et al. "Increased cutaneous nerve fibers in female specimens." *Plastic and Reconstructive Surgery* 116, no. 5 (2005): 1407-10.

8. Vincent K, Warnaby C, Stagg CJ, et al. "Dysmenorrhoea is associated with central changes in otherwise healthy women." *Pain* 152, no. 9 (2011): 1966-75; Sarajari S, Oblinger MM. "Estrogen effects on pain sensitivity and neuropeptide expression in rat sensory neurons." *Experimental Neurology* 224, no. 1 (2010): 163-69.

9. National Institute of Neurological Disorders and Stroke. "Pain: Hope through research." www.ninds.nih.gov/disorders/chronic_pain/detail_chronic_pain.htm.

10. Lew HL, Otis JD, Tun C, et al. "Prevalence of chronic pain, posttraumatic stress disorder, and persistent postconcussive symptoms in OIF/OEF veterans: Polytrauma clinical triad." *Journal of Rehabilitation Research & Development* 46, no. 6 (2009): 697-702; Beckham JC, Crawford AL, Feldman ME, "Chronic posttraumatic stress disorder and chronic pain in Vietnam combat veterans." *Journal of Psychosomatic Research* 43, no. 4 (1997): 379-89.

11. Theeler BJ, Flynn FG, Erickson JC. "Chronic daily headache in U.S. soldiers after concussion." *Headache* 52, no. 5 (2012): 732-38.

Chapter 2. Chronically Painful Conditions

1. Sawitzke AD, Shi H, Finco MF, et al. "The effect of glucosamine and/or chondroitin of sulfate on the progression of knee osteoarthritis: A report from the glucosamine/chondroitin arthritis intervention trial." *Arthritis and Rheumatism* 58, no. 10 (2008): 3183-91.

2. Van den Beuken-van Everdingen MH, de Rijke JM, Kessels AG, et al. "Prevalence of pain in patients with cancer: A systematic review of the past 40 years." *Annals of Oncology* 18, no. 9 (2007): 1437-49; Pharo GH, Zhou L. "Pharmacologic management of cancer pain." *Journal of the American Osteopathic Association* 105, suppl 5 (2005): S21-S28.

3. Sarchielli P, Mancini ML, Floridi A, et al. "Increased levels of neurotrophins are not specific for chronic migraine: Evidence from primary fibromyalgia syndrome." *Journal of Pain* 8, no. 9 (2007): 737-45; Vaerøy H, Helle R, Førre O, et al. "Elevated CSF levels of substance P and high incidence of Raynaud phenomenon in patients with fibromyalgia: New features for diagnosis." *Pain* 32, no. 1 (1988): 21-26; Russell IJ, Orr MD, Littman B, et al. "Elevated cerebrospinal levels of substance P in patients with the fibromyalgia syndrome." *Arthritis and Rheumatism* 37, no. 11 (1994): 1593-1601.

4. Brosseau L, Wells GA, Tugwell P, et al. "Ottawa Panel evidence-based clinical practice guidelines for aerobic fitness exercises in the management of fibromyalgia: Part 1." *Physical Therapy* 88, no. 7 (2008): 857-71; Brosseau L, Wells GA, Tugwell P, et al. "Ottawa Panel evidence-based clinical practice guidelines for strengthening exercises in the management of fibromyalgia: Part 2." *Physical Therapy* 88, no. 7 (2008): 873-86.

5. Juliano LM, Griffiths RR. "A critical review of caffeine withdrawal: Empirical validation of symptoms and signs, incidence, severity, and associated features." *Psychopharmacology* 176, no. 1 (2004): 1-29.

6. Aurora SK, Winner P, Freeman MC, et al. "OnabotulinumtoxinA for treatment of

chronic migraine: Pooled analyses of the 56-Week PREEMPT clinical program." *Headache* 51, no. 9 (2011): 1358-73.

7. Weinstein JN, Lurie JD, Tosteson TD, et al. "Surgery vs. nonoperative treatment for lumbar disk herniation: The Spine Patient Outcomes Research Trial (SPORT): A randomized trial." *Journal of the American Medical Association* 296, no. 20 (2006): 2441-50; Weinstein JN, Tosteson TD, Lurie JD, et al. "Surgical versus nonoperative treatment for lumbar spinal stenosis: Four-year results of the Spine Patient Outcomes Research Trial." *Spine* 35, no. 14 (2010): 1329-38; Weinstein JN, Lurie JD, Tosteson TD, et al. "Surgical compared with nonoperative treatment for lumbar degenerative spondylolisthesis: Four-year results in the Spine Patient Outcomes Research Trial (SPORT) randomized and observational cohorts." *Journal of Bone and Joint Surgery* 91, no. 6 (2009): 1295-1304.

8. Yanow J, Pappagallo M, Pillai L. "Complex regional pain syndrome (CRPS/RSD) and neuropathic pain: Role of intravenous bisphosphonates as analgesics." *Scientific World Journal* 8 (2008): 229-36; Goldberg ME, Torjman MC, Schwartzman RJ, et al. "Pharmacodynamic profiles of ketamine (R)- and (S)- with 5-day inpatient infusion for the treatment of complex regional pain syndrome." *Pain Physician* 13, no. 4 (2010): 379-87; Schwartzman RJ, Alexander GM, Grothusen JR, et al. "Outpatient intravenous ketamine for the treatment of complex regional pain syndrome: A double-blind placebo controlled study." *Pain* 147, nos. 1-3 (2009): 107-15.

9. Anderson RU, Wise D, Sawyer T, et al. "6-day intensive treatment protocol for refractory chronic prostatitis/chronic pelvic pain syndrome using myofascial release and paradoxical relaxation training." *Journal of Urology* 185, no. 4 (2011): 1294-99.

10. Karanikolas M, Aretha D, Tsolakis I, et al. "Optimized perioperative analgesia reduces chronic phantom limb pain intensity, prevalence, and frequency: A prospective, randomized, clinical trial." *Anesthesiology* 114, no. 5 (2011): 1144-54.

11. Ramachandran VS, Rogers-Ramachandran D. "Synaesthesia in phantom limbs induced with mirrors." *Proceedings: Biological Sciences* 263, no. 1369 (1996): 377-86; Cacchio A, De Blasis E, Necozione S, et al. "Mirror therapy for chronic complex regional pain syndrome type 1 and stroke." *New England Journal of Medicine* 361, no. 6 (2009): 634-36.

12. Frissora CL, Koch KL. "Symptom overlap and comorbidity of irritable bowel syndrome with other conditions." *Current Gastroenterology Reports* 7, no. 4 (2004): 264-71; Chia JK, Chia AY. "Chronic fatigue syndrome is associated with chronic enterovirus infection of the stomach." *Journal of Clinical Pathology* 61, no. 1 (2008): 43-48.

13. Lerner AM, Beqaj S, Fitzgerald JT, et al. "Subset-directed antiviral treatment of 142 herpesvirus patients with chronic fatigue syndrome." *Virus Adaptation and Treatment* 2 (2010): 47-57.

Chapter 3. Pain Medications and How They Work

1. Fosbøl EL, Folke F, Jacobsen S, et al. "Cause-specific cardiovascular risk associated with nonsteroidal anti-inflammatory drugs among healthy individuals." *Circulation* 3, no. 4 (2010): 395-405; Shau WY, Chen HC, Chen ST, et al. "Risk of new acute myocardial infarction hospitalization associated with use of oral and parenteral non-steroidal anti-inflammation drugs (NSAIDs): A case-crossover study of Taiwan's National Health Insur-

ance claims database and review of current evidence." *BMC Cardiovascular Disorders* 12, no. 4 (2012), www.biomedcentral.com/1471-2261/12/4.

2. Olsen A-M, Fosbøl EL, Lindhardsen J, et al. "Long-term cardiovascular risk of NSAID use according to time passed after first-time myocardial infarction: A nationwide cohort study." *Circulation* 126, no. 16 (October 16, 2012): 1955-63.

3. Laine L, Kivitz AJ, Bello AE, et al. "Double-blind randomized trials of single-tablet ibuprofen/high-dose famotidine vs. ibuprofen alone for reduction of gastric and duodenal ulcers." *American Journal of Gastroenterology* 107, no. 3 (2012): 379-86.

4. Malinoff HL, Barkin RL, Wilson G. "Sublingual buprenorphine is effective in the treatment of chronic pain syndrome." *American Journal of Therapeutics* 12, no. 5 (2005): 379-84; Wolff RF, Aune D, Truyers C, et al. "Systematic review of efficacy and safety of buprenorphine versus fentanyl or morphine in patients with chronic moderate to severe pain." *Current Medical Research and Opinion* 28, no 5 (2012): 833-45.

5. Centers for Disease Control and Prevention. "Prescription painkiller overdoses in the U.S." www.cdc.gov/vitalsigns/PainkillerOverdoses.

6. National Institutes for Health. "Opioids and chronic pain." www.nlm.nih.gov/medlineplus/magazine/issues/spring11/articles/spring11pg9.html.

7. Noble M, Treadwell JR, Tregear SJ, et al. "Long-term opioid management for chronic noncancer pain." *Cochrane Database System Reviews* 2010 (1): CD006605.

8. Mitchell JM, Basbaum AI, Fields HL. "A locus and mechanism of action for associative morphine tolerance." *Nature and Neuroscience* 3, no. 1 (2000): 47-53.

9. Bingel U, Wanigasekera V, Wiech K, et al. "The effect of treatment expectation on drug efficacy: Imaging the analgesic benefit of the opioid remifentanil." *Science Translational Medicine* 3, no. 70 (2011): 70ra14.

10. Urquhart DM, Hoving JL, Assendelft WW, et al. "Antidepressants for non-specific low-back pain." *Cochrane Database of Systematic Reviews* 1 (2008): CD001703.

11. Hochberg MC, Wohlreich M, Gaynor P, et al. "Clinically relevant outcomes based on analysis of pooled data from 2 trials of duloxetine in patients with knee osteoarthritis." *Journal of Rheumatology* 39, no. 2 (2012): 352-58.

12. Frakes EP, Risser RC, Ball TD, et al. "Duloxetine added to oral nonsteroidal anti-inflammatory drugs for treatment of knee pain due to osteoarthritis: Results of a randomized, double-blind, placebo-controlled trial." *Current Medical Research and Opinion* 27, no. 12 (2011): 2361-72.

13. Pergolizzi JV Jr, Raffa RB, Taylor R Jr, et al. "A review of duloxetine 60 mg once-daily dosing for the management of diabetic peripheral neuropathic pain, fibromyalgia, and chronic musculoskeletal pain due to chronic osteoarthritis pain and low back pain." *Pain Practice,* June 21, 2012. doi: 10.1111/j.1533-2500.2012.00578.x.

14. Hocking G, Cousins MJ. "Ketamine in chronic pain management: An evidence-based review." *Anesthesia and Analgesia* 97, no. 6 (2003): 1730-39.

15. Schwartzman RJ, Alexander GM, Grothusen JR, et al. "Outpatient intravenous ketamine for the treatment of complex regional pain syndrome: A double-blind placebo controlled study." *Pain* 147, nos. 1-3 (2009): 107-15; Sigtermans MJ, van Hilten JJ, Bauer MC, et al. "Ketamine produces effective and long-term pain relief in patients with Complex Regional Pain Syndrome Type 1." *Pain* 145, no. 3 (2009): 304-11; Subramaniam K, Subra-

maniam B, Steinbrook RA. "Ketamine as adjuvant analgesic to opioids: A quantitative and qualitative systematic review." *Anesthesia and Analgesia* 99, no. 2 (2004): 482-95.

16. Nikolajsen L, Gottrup H, Kristensen AG, et al. "Memantine (a *N*-methyl-D-aspartate receptor antagonist) in the treatment of neuropathic pain after amputation or surgery: A randomized, double-blinded, cross-over study." *Anesthesia and Analgesia* 91, no. 4 (2000): 960-66; Schifitto G, Yiannoutsos CT, Simpson DM, et al. "A placebo-controlled study of memantine for the treatment of human immunodeficiency virus-associated sensory neuropathy." *Journal of Neurovirology* 12, no. 4 (2006): 328-31.

17. Goebel A, Baranowski A, Maurer K, et al. "Intravenous immunoglobulin treatment of the complex regional pain syndrome: A randomized trial." *Annals of Internal Medicine* 152, no 3 (2010): 152-58.

18. Richards BL, Whittle SL, Buchbinder R. "Muscle relaxants for pain management in rheumatoid arthritis." *Cochrane Database of Systematic Reviews* 1 (2012): CD008922.

19. Narang S, Gibson D, Wasan AD, et al. "Efficacy of dronabinol as an adjuvant treatment for chronic pain patients on opioid therapy." *Journal of Pain* 9, no. 3 (2008): 254-64.

20. Rog DJ, Nurmikko TJ, Friede T, et al. "Randomized, controlled trial of cannabis-based medicine in central pain in multiple sclerosis." *Neurology* 65, no. 6 (2005): 812-19; Zajicek JP, Hobart JC, Slade A, et al. "Multiple sclerosis and extract of cannabis: Results of the MUSEC trial." *Journal of Neurology, Neurosurgery, and Psychiatry* 83, no. 11 (2012): 1125-32.

21. Institute of Medicine. *Marijuana and Medicine: Assessing the Science Base.* Washington, DC: National Academy Press, 1999:141; Raft D, Gregg J, Ghia J, et al. "Effects of intravenous tetrahydrocannabinol on experimental and surgical pain: Psychological correlates of the analgesic response." *Clinical Pharmacology and Therapeutics* 21, no. 1 (1977): 26-33.

Chapter 4. Mind-over-Pain Therapies

1. Lamé IE, Peters ML, Viaeyen JW, et al. "Quality of life in chronic pain is more associated with beliefs about pain, than with pain intensity." *European Journal of Pain* 9, no. 1 (2005): 15-24.

2. Goffaux P, de Souza JB, Potvin S, et al. "Pain relief through expectation supersedes descending inhibitory deficits in fibromyalgia patients." *Pain* 145, nos. 1-2 (2009): 18-23.

3. Bingel U, Wanigasekera V, Wiech K, et al. "The effect of treatment expectation on drug efficacy: Imaging the analgesic benefit of the opioid Remifentanil." *Science Translational Medicine* 3, no. 70 (2011): 70ra14.

4. Koyama T, McHaffie JG, Laurienti PJ, et al. "The subjective experience of pain: Where expectations become reality." *Proceedings of the National Academy of Sciences of the United States of America* 102, no. 36 (2005): 12950-55; Sawamoto N, Honda M, Okada T, et al. "Expectation of pain enhances responses to nonpainful somatosensory stimulation in the anterior cingulate cortex and parietal operculum/posterior insula: An event-related functional magnetic resonance imaging study." *Journal of Neuroscience* 20, no. 19 (2000): 7438-45; Villemure C, Bushnell MC. "Mood influences supraspinal pain processing separately from attention." *Journal of Neuroscience* 29, no. 3 (2009): 705-15.

5. Duncan GH, Bushnell MC, Bates R, et al. "Task-related responses of monkey medullary dorsal horn neurons." *Journal of Neurophysiology* 57, no. 1 (1987): 289-310.

6. Corradi-Dell'Acqua C, Hofstetter C, Vuilleumier P. "Felt and seen pain evoke the same local patterns of cortical activity in insular and cingulate cortex." *Journal of Neuroscience* 31, no. 49 (2011): 17996-18006; Seifert F, Schuberth N, De Col R, et al. "Brain activity during sympathetic response in anticipation and experience of pain." *Human Brain Mapping* 2012 Mar 22. doi: 10.1002/hbm.22035.

7. Gaylord SA, Palsson OS, Garland EL, et al. "Mindfulness training reduces the severity of irritable bowel syndrome in women: Results of a randomized controlled trial." *American Journal of Gastroenterology* 106, no. 9 (2011): 1678-88; Rosenzweig S, Greeson JM, Reibel DK, et al. "Mindfulness-based stress reduction for chronic pain conditions: Variation in treatment outcomes and role of home meditation practice." *Journal of Psychosomatic Research* 68, no. 1 (2010): 29-36.

8. Goossens ME, Vlaeyen JW, Hidding A, et al. "Treatment expectancy affects the outcome of cognitive-behavioral interventions in chronic pain." *Clinical Journal of Pain* 21, no. 1 (2005): 18-26.

9. Derbyshire SW, Whalley MG, Oakley DA. "Fibromyalgia pain and its modulation by hypnotic and non-hypnotic suggestion: An fMRI analysis." *European Journal of Pain* 13, no. 5 (2009): 542-50; Emami MH, Gholamrezaei A, Daneshgar H. "Hypnotherapy as an adjuvant for the management of inflammatory bowel disease: A case report." *American Journal of Clinical Hypnosis* 51, no. 3 (2009): 255-62.

10. Elkins G, Jensen MP, Patterson DR. "Hypnotherapy for the management of chronic pain." *International Journal of Clinical and Experimental Hypnosis* 55, no. 3 (2007): 275-87.

11. Dunbar RI, Baron R, Frangou A, et al. "Social laughter is correlated with an elevated pain threshold." *Proceedings of the Royal Society B: Biological Sciences* 279, no. 1731 (2012): 1161-67.

Chapter 5. Body-over-Pain Therapies

1. Kelley GA, Kelley KS, Hootman JM, et al. "Effects of community-deliverable exercise on pain and physical function in adults with arthritis and other rheumatic diseases: A meta-analysis." *Arthritis Care and Research* 63, no. 1 (2011): 79-93.

2. Wong P, Muanza T, Hijal T, et al. "Effect of exercise in reducing breast and chest-wall pain in patients with breast cancer: A pilot study." *Current Oncology* 19, no. 3 (2012): e129-35.

3. Buenaver LF, Quartana PJ, Grace EG, et al. "Evidence for indirect effects of pain catastrophizing on clinical pain among myofascial temporomandibular disorder participants: The mediating role of sleep disturbance." *Pain* 153, no. 6 (2012): 1159-66.

4. Dyson-Hudson TA, Shiflett SC, Kirshblum SC, et al. "Acupuncture and Trager psychophysical integration in the treatment of wheelchair user's shoulder pain in individuals with spinal cord injury." *Archives of Physical Medicine and Rehabilitation* 82, no. 8 (2001): 1038-46.

5. Little P, Lewith G, Webley F, et al. "Randomised controlled trial of Alexander technique lessons, exercise, and massage (ATEAM) for chronic and recurrent back pain." *British Journal of Sports Medicine* 42, no. 12 (2008): 965-68.

6. Flegal KM, Carroll MD, Ogden CL, et al. "Prevalence and trends in obesity among U.S. adults, 1999-2008." *Journal of the American Medical Association* 303, no. 3 (2010): 235-41.

7. Samartzis D, Karppinen J, Chan D, et al. "The association of lumbar intervertebral disc degeneration on magnetic resonance imaging with body mass index in overweight and obese adults: A population-based study." *Arthritis and Rheumatism* 64, no. 5 (2012): 1488-96.

8. Kim CH, Luedtke CA, Vincent A, et al. "Association of body mass index with symptom severity and quality of life in patients with fibromyalgia." *Arthritis Care and Research* 64, no. 2 (2012): 222-28.

9. Stone AA, Broderick JE. "Obesity and pain are associated in the United States." *Obesity* 20, no. 7 (2012): 1491-95.

10. Lin JS, O'Connor E, Whitlock EP, et al. "Behavioral counseling to promote physical activity and a healthful diet to prevent cardiovascular disease in adults: Systematic review for the U.S. Preventive Services Task Force." *Annals of Internal Medicine* 153, no. 11 (2010): 736-50.

11. Galarraga B, Ho M, Youssef HM, et al. "Cod liver oil (n-3 fatty acids) as an nonsteroidal anti-inflammatory drug sparing agent in rheumatoid arthritis." *Rheumatology* 47, no. 5 (2008): 665-69.

12. Ibid.; Kremer JM. "N-3 fatty acid supplements in rheumatoid arthritis." *American Journal of Clinical Nutrition* 71, no. 1 suppl (2000): 349s-51s.

13. Knott L, Avery NC, Hollander AP, et al. "Regulation of osteoarthritis by omega-3 (n-3) polyunsaturated fatty acids in a naturally occurring model of disease." *Osteoarthritis and Cartilage* 19, no. 9 (2011): 1150-57; Maroon JC, Bost JW. "Omega-3 fatty acids (fish oil) as an anti-inflammatory: An alternative to nonsteroidal anti-inflammatory drugs for discogenic pain." *Surgical Neurology* 65, no. 4 (2006): 326-31.

14. Lopez-Garcia E, Schulze MB, Meigs JB, et al. "Consumption of trans fatty acids is related to plasma biomarkers of inflammation and endothelial dysfunction." *Journal of Nutrition* 135, no. 3 (2005): 562-66.

15. Choi HK, Atkinson K, Karlson EW, et al. "Purine-rich foods, dairy and protein intake, and the risk of gout in men." *New England Journal of Medicine* 350 (2004): 1093-1103.

16. Choi HK, Atkinson K, Karlson EW, et al. "Alcohol intake and risk of incident gout in men: A prospective study." *Lancet* 363, no. 9417 (2004): 1277-81.

17. Choi HK, Curhan G. "Soft drinks, fructose consumption, and the risk of gout in men: Prospective cohort study." *British Medical Journal* 336, no. 7639 (2008): 309-12.

18. Holton KF, Taren DL, Thomson CA, et al. "The effect of dietary glutamate on fibromyalgia and irritable bowel symptoms." *Clinical and Experimental Rheumatology* 30, no. 6, suppl. 74 (November-December 2012): 10-17.

19. Hirani V. "Vitamin D status and pain: Analysis from the Health Survey for England among English adults aged 65 years and over." *British Journal of Nutrition* 107, no. 7 (2012): 1080-84; Abokrysha NT. "Vitamin D deficiency in women with fibromyalgia in Saudi Arabia." *Pain Medicine* 13, no. 3 (2012): 452-58; Matthana MH. "The relation between vitamin D deficiency and fibromyalgia syndrome in women." *Saudi Medical Journal* 32, no. 9 (2011): 925-29.

20. Turner MK, Hooten WM, Schmidt JE, et al. "Prevalence and clinical correlates of vitamin D inadequacy among patients with chronic pain." *Pain Medicine* 9, no. 8 (2008): 979-84.

21. Demirkaya S, Vural O, Dora B, et al. "Efficacy of intravenous magnesium sulfate in the treatment of acute migraine attacks." *Headache* 41, no. 2 (2001): 171-77; Collins S, Zuurmond WW, de Lange JJ, et al. "Intravenous magnesium for complex regional pain syndrome type 1 (CRPS 1) patients: A pilot study." *Pain Medicine* 10, no. 5 (2009): 930-40; Brill S, Sedgwick PM, Hamann W, et al. "Efficacy of intravenous magnesium in neuropathic pain." *British Journal of Anaesthesia* 89, no. 5 (2002): 711-14.

22. Kim DJ, Xun P, Liu K, et al. "Magnesium intake in relation to systemic inflammation, insulin resistance, and the incidence of diabetes." *Diabetes Care* 33, no. 12 (2010): 2604-10.

23. Abraham GE, Flechas JD. "Management of fibromyalgia: Rationale for the use of magnesium and malic acid." *Journal of Nutritional and Environmental Medicine* 3, no. 1 (1992): 49-59; Russell IJ, Michalek JE, Flechas JD, et al. "Treatment of fibromyalgia syndrome with Super Malic: A randomized, double blind, placebo controlled, crossover pilot study." *Journal of Rheumatology* 22, no. 5 (1995): 953-58; Bagis S, Karabiber M, As I, et al. "Is magnesium citrate treatment effective on pain, clinical parameters and functional status in patients with fibromyalgia?" *Rheumatology International* 2012 Jan 22. doi: 10.1007/s00296-011-2334-8.

24. Dagenais S, Yelland MJ, Del Mar C, et al. "Prolotherapy injections for chronic low-back pain." *Cochrane Database of Systematic Reviews* 18, no. 2 (2007): CD004059.

25. Johnson M, Martinson M. "Efficacy of electrical nerve stimulation for chronic musculoskeletal pain: A meta-analysis of randomized controlled trials." *Pain* 130, nos. 1-2 (2007): 157-65.

26. Rasche D, Rinaldi PC, Young RF, et al. "Deep brain stimulation for the treatment of various chronic pain syndromes." *Neurosurgical Focus* 21, no. 6 (2006): E8; Bittar RG, Kar-Purkayastha I, Owen SL, et al. "Deep brain stimulation for pain relief: A meta-analysis." *Journal of Clinical Neuroscience* 12, no. 5 (2005): 515-19.

27. Khedr E, Kotb H, Kamel N, et al. "Longlasting antalgic effects of daily sessions of repetitive transcranial magnetic stimulation in central and peripheral neuropathic pain." *Journal of Neurology, Neurosurgery, and Psychiatry* 76, no. 6 (2005): 833-38; Smania N, Corato E, Fiaschi A, et al. "Repetitive magnetic stimulation: A novel therapeutic approach for myofascial pain syndrome." *Journal of Neurology* 252, no. 3 (2005): 307-14.

Chapter 6. Complementary and Alternative Therapies

1. Dorsher PT. "Myofascial referred-pain data provide physiologic evidence of acupuncture meridians." *Journal of Pain* 10, no. 7 (2009): 723-31.

2. Ritenbaugh C, Hammerschlag R, Dworkin SF, et al. "Comparative effectiveness of traditional Chinese medicine and psychosocial care in the treatment of temporomandibular disorders-associated chronic facial pain." *Journal of Pain* 13, no. 11 (2012): 1075-89.

3. Zencirci B, Yuksel KZ, Gumusalan Y. "Effectiveness of acupuncture with NSAID medication in the management of acute discogenic radicular pain: A randomised, controlled trial." *Journal of Anesthesia and Clinical Research* 3, no. 203 (2012). doi: 10.4172/2155-6148.1000203, www.omicsonline.org/2155-6148/2155-6148- 3-203.php?aid=5974.

4. Qu M, Ding XN, Liu HB, et al. "Clinical observation on acupuncture combined with

nerve block for treatment of lumbar disc herniation." *Chinese Acupuncture and Moxibustion* 30, no. 8 (2010): 633-36.

5. Schröder S, Liepert J, Remppis A, et al. "Acupuncture treatment improves nerve conduction in peripheral neuropathy." *European Journal of Neurology* 14, no. 3 (2007): 276-81.

6. Ahn AC, Bennani T, Freeman R, et al. "Two styles of acupuncture for treating painful diabetic neuropathy—a pilot randomised control trial." *Acupuncture in Medicine* 25, nos. 1-2 (2007): 11-17.

7. Ernst E, Lee MS, Choi T. "Acupuncture: Does it alleviate pain and are there serious risks? A review of reviews." *Pain* 152, no. 4 (2011): 755-64; Linde K, Allais G, Brinkhaus B, et al. "Acupuncture for migraine prophylaxis." *Cochrane Database of Systematic Reviews* 21, no. 1 (2009): CD001218; Li Y, Zheng H, Witt CM, et al. "Acupuncture for migraine prophylaxis: A randomized controlled trial." *Canadian Medical Association Journal* 184, no. 4 (2012): 401-10.

8. Matsubara T, Arai YC, Shiro Y, et al. "Comparative effects of acupressure at local and distal acupuncture points on pain conditions and autonomic function in females with chronic neck pain." *Evidence-Based Complementary and Alternative Medicine*. Published online 2011 (2011). doi: 10.1155/2011/543291.

9. Robinson N, Lorenc A, Liao X. "The evidence for Shiatsu: A systematic review of Shiatsu and acupressure." *BMC Complementary and Alternative Medicine* 11 (2011): 88.

10. Ross A, Thomas S. "The health benefits of yoga and exercise: A review of comparison studies." *Journal of Alternative and Complementary Medicine* 16, no. 1 (2010): 3-12.

11. Sherman KJ, Cherkin DC, Wellman RD, et al. "A randomized trial comparing yoga, stretching, and a self-care book for chronic low back pain." *Archives of Internal Medicine* 171, no. 22 (2011): 2019-26.

12. Williams K, Abildso C, Steinberg L, et al. "Evaluation of the effectiveness and efficacy of Iyengar yoga therapy on chronic low back pain." *Spine* 34, no. 19 (2009): 2066-76; Tilbrook HE, Cox H, Hewitt CE, et al. "Yoga for chronic low back pain: A randomized trial." *Annals of Internal Medicine* 155, no. 9 (2011): 569-78.

13. Curtis K, Osadchuk A, Katz J. "An eight-week yoga intervention is associated with improvements in pain, psychological functioning and mindfulness, and changes in cortisol levels in women with fibromyalgia." *Journal of Pain Research* no. 4 (2011): 189-201; Carson JW, Carson KM, Jones KD, et al. "A pilot randomized controlled trial of the Yoga of Awareness program in the management of fibromyalgia." *Pain* 151, no. 2 (2010): 530-39.

14. Irwin MR, Olmstead R, Oxman MN. "Augmenting immune responses to varicella zoster virus in older adults: A randomized, controlled trial of tai chi." *Journal of the American Geriatrics Society* 55, no. 4 (2007): 511-17; Yeh GY, Wang C, Wayne PM, et al. "The effect of tai chi exercise on blood pressure: A systematic review." *Preventive Cardiology* 11, no. 2 (2008): 82-89; Jahnke R, Larkey L, Rogers C, et al. "A comprehensive review of health benefits of qigong and tai chi." *American Journal of Health Promotion* 24, no. 6 (2010): e1-e25.

15. Field T. "Tai chi research review." *Complementary Therapies in Clinical Practice* 17, no. 3 (2011): 141-46; Wang C, Schmid CH, Rones R, et al. "A randomized trial of tai chi

for fibromyalgia." *New England Journal of Medicine* 363, no. 8 (2010): 743-54; Jones KD, Sherman CA, Mist SD, et al. "A randomized controlled trial of 8-form tai chi improves symptoms and functional mobility in fibromyalgia patients." *Clinical Rheumatology* 31, no. 8 (2012): 1205-14; Lee HY, Hale CA, Hemingway B, et al. "Tai chi exercise and auricular acupressure for people with rheumatoid arthritis: An evaluation study." *Journal of Clinical Nursing* 21, nos. 19-20 (2012): 2812-22.

16. Lee MS, Pittler MH, Ernst E. "Tai chi for osteoarthritis: A systematic review." *Clinical Rheumatology* 27, no. 2 (2008): 211-18.

17. Wajswelner H, Metcalf B, Bennell K. "Clinical Pilates versus general exercise for chronic low back pain: Randomized trial." *Medicine and Science in Sports and Exercise* 44, no. 7 (2012): 1197-1205.

18. Dyson-Hudson TA, Shiflett SC, Kirshblum SC, et al. "Acupuncture and Trager psychophysical integration in the treatment of wheelchair user's shoulder pain in individuals with spinal cord injury." *Archives of Physical Medicine and Rehabilitation* 82, no. 8 (2001): 1038-46.

19. Ohman A, Aström L, Malmgren-Olsson EB. "Feldenkrais therapy as group treatment for chronic pain—a qualitative evaluation." *Journal of Bodywork and Movement Therapies* 15, no. 2 (2011): 153-61.

20. Sima AA, Calvani M, Mehra M, et al. "acetyl-L-carnitine improves pain, nerve regeneration, and vibratory perception in patients with chronic diabetic neuropathy: An analysis of two randomized placebo-controlled trials." *Diabetes Care* 28, no. 1 (2005): 89-94.

21. Ross SM. "Osteoarthritis: A proprietary arnica gel is found to be as effective as ibuprofen gel in osteoarthritis of the hands." *Holistic Nursing Practice* 22, no. 4 (2008): 237-39; Widrig R, Suter A, Saller R, et al. "Choosing between NSAID and arnica for topical treatment of hand osteoarthritis in a randomized, double-blind study." *Rheumatology International* 27, no. 6 (2007): 585-91; Knuesel O, Weber M, Suter A. "Arnica montana gel in osteoarthritis of the knee: An open, multicenter clinical trial." *Advances in Therapy* 19, no. 5 (2002): 209-18.

22. Brendler T, Gruenwald J, Ulbricht C, et al. "Devil's claw (harpagophytum procumbens DC): An evidence-based systematic review by the Natural Standard Research Collaboration." *Journal of Herbal Pharmacotherapy* 6, no. 1 (2006): 89-126; Brien S, Lewith GT, McGregor G. "Devil's claw (harpagophytum procumbens) as a treatment for osteoarthritis: A review of efficacy and safety." *Journal of Alternative and Complementary Medicine* 12, no. 10 (2006): 981-93.

23. Chrubasik JE, Roufogalis BD, Chrubasik S. "Evidence of effectiveness of herbal antiinflammatory drugs in the treatment of painful osteoarthritis and chronic low back pain." *Phytotherapy Research* 21, no. 7 (2007): 675-83; Drozdov VN, Kim VA, Tkachenko EV, et al. "Influence of a specific ginger combination on gastropathy conditions in patients with osteoarthritis of the knee or hip." *Journal of Alternative and Complementary Medicine* 18, no. 6 (2012): 583-88.

24. Halat KM, Dennehy CE. "Botanicals and dietary supplements in diabetic peripheral neuropathy." *Journal of the American Board of Family Practice* 16, no. 1 (2003): 47-57; Belch JJ, Hill A. "Evening primrose oil and borage oil in rheumatologic conditions." *Amer-*

ican Journal of Clinical Nutrition 71, no. 1 suppl (2000): 352S-56S; Keen H, Payan J, Allawi J, et al. "Treatment of diabetic neuropathy with gamma-linolenic acid: The Gamma-Linolenic Acid Multicenter Trial Group." *Diabetes Care* 16, no. 1 (1993): 8-15.

25. Vanderpool C, Yan F, Polk DB. "Mechanisms of probiotic action: Implications for therapeutic applications in inflammatory bowel diseases." *Inflammatory Bowel Diseases* 14, no. 11 (2008): 1585-96.

26. Zhang R-X, Fan AY, Zhou A-N, et al. "Extract of the Chinese herbal formula *Huo Luo Xiao Ling Dan* inhibited adjuvant arthritis in rats." *Journal of Ethnopharmacology* 121, no. 3 (2009): 366-71.

27. "Fragrance reduces migraines." Smell and Taste Treatment and Research Foundation. www.smellandtaste.org.

28. Kiecolt-Glaser JK, Graham JE, Malarkey WB, et al. "Olfactory influences on mood and autonomic, endocrine, and immune function." *Psychoneuroendocrinology* 33, no. 3 (2008): 328-39.

29. Lua PL, Zakaria NS. "A brief review of current scientific evidence involving aromatherapy use for nausea and vomiting." *Journal of Alternative and Complementary Medicine* 18, no. 6 (2012): 534-40.

30. Furst DE, Venkatraman MM, McGann M, et al. "Double-blind, randomized, controlled, pilot study comparing classic Ayurvedic medicine, methotrexate, and their combination in rheumatoid arthritis." *Journal of Clinical Rheumatology* 17, no. 4 (2011): 185-92.

31. Saper RB, Phillips RS, Sehgal A, et al. "Lead, mercury, and arsenic in U.S. and Indian-manufactured Ayurvedic medicines sold via the Internet." *Journal of the American Medical Association* 300, no. 8 (2008): 915-23.

Chapter 7. Spirit over Pain

1. McCord G, Gilchrist VJ, Grossman SD, et al. "Discussing spirituality with patients: A rational and ethical approach." *Annals of Family Medicine* 2, no. 4 (2004): 356-61.

2. Williams JA, Meltzer D, Arora V, et al. "Attention to inpatients' religious and spiritual concerns: Predictors and association with patient satisfaction." *Journal of General Internal Medicine* 26, no. 11 (2011): 1265-71.

3. Dunn KS, Horgas AL. "Religious and nonreligious coping in older adults experiencing chronic pain." *Pain Management Nursing* 5, no. 1 (2004): 19-28; Glover-Graf N, Marini I, Buck T. "Religious and spiritual beliefs and practices of persons with chronic pain." *Rehabilitation Counseling Bulletin* 51, no. 1 (2007): 21-33.

4. Pargament KI, Smith BW, Koenig HG, et al. "Patterns of positive and negative religious coping with major life stressors." *Journal for the Scientific Study of Religion* 37, no. 4 (1998): 710-24.

5. Glazer S. "Can spirituality influence health?" *Prayer and Healing* 15, no. 2 (2005): 1-35.

6. Wachholtz A, Sambamoorthi U. "National trends in prayer use as a coping mechanism for health concerns: Changes from 2002 to 2007." *Psychology of Religion and Spirituality* 3, no. 2 (2011): 67-77.

7. Shi Q, Langer G, Cohen J, et al. "People in pain: How do they seek relief?" *Journal of Pain* 8, no. 8 (2007): 624-36.

8. Perlman DM, Salomons TV, Davidson RJ, et al. "Differential effects on pain intensity and unpleasantness of two meditation practices." *Emotion* 10, no. 1 (2010): 65-71.

9. Wachholtz AB, Pargament KI. "Is spirituality a critical ingredient of meditation? Comparing the effects of spiritual meditation, secular meditation, and relaxation on spiritual, psychological, cardiac, and pain outcomes." *Journal of Behavioral Medicine* 28, no. 4 (2005): 369-84; Wachholtz AB, Pargament KI. "Migraines and meditation: Does spirituality matter?" *Journal of Behavioral Medicine* 31, no. 4 (2008): 351-66.

10. Wood AM, Joseph S, Maltby J. "Gratitude predicts psychological well-being above the Big Five facets." *Personality and Individual Differences* 46, no 4 (2009): 443-47.

11. Wood AM, Joseph S, Lloyd J, et al. "Gratitude influences sleep through the mechanism of pre-sleep cognitions." *Journal of Psychosomatic Research* 66, no. 1 (2009): 43-48.

Chapter 8. The Family in Pain

1. Leong LE, Cano A, Johansen AB. "Sequential and base rate analysis of emotional validation and invalidation in chronic pain couples: Patient gender matters." *Journal of Pain* 12, no. 11 (2011): 1140-48.

2. Cano A, Leong L, Heller JB, et al. "Perceived entitlement to pain-related support and pain catastrophizing: Associations with perceived and observed support." *Pain* 147, nos. 1-3 (2009): 249-54.

Chapter 10. The Future of Pain Management

1. Wang X, Loram LC, Ramos K, et al. "Morphine activates neuroinflammation in a manner parallel to endotoxin." *Proceedings of the National Academy of Sciences of the United States of America* 109, no. 16 (2012): 6325-30.

2. Wiley RG, Kline RH IV, Vierck CJ Jr. "Anti-nociceptive effects of selectively destroying substance P receptor-expressing dorsal horn neurons using [Sar9, Met (O2)11]-substance P-saporin: Behavioral and anatomical analyses." *Neuroscience* 146, no. 3 (2007): 1333-45.

3. Kohr D, Singh P, Tschernatsch M, et al. "Autoimmunity against the β2 adrenergic receptor and muscarinic-2 receptor in complex regional pain syndrome." *Pain* 152, no. 12 (2011): 2690-700; Goebel A, Baranowski A, Maurer K, et al. "Intravenous immunoglobulin treatment of the complex regional pain syndrome: A randomized trial." *Annals of Internal Medicine* 152, no. 3 (2010): 152-58.

4. Picarelli H, Teixeira MJ, de Andrade DC, et al. "Repetitive transcranial magnetic stimulation is efficacious as an add-on to pharmacological therapy in complex regional pain syndrome (CRPS) type I." *Journal of Pain* 11, no. 11 (2010): 1203-10.

5. Marlow NM, Bonilha HS, Short EB. "Efficacy of transcranial direct current stimulation and repetitive transcranial magnetic stimulation for treating fibromyalgia syndrome: A systematic review." *Pain Practice,* May 28, 2012. doi: 10.1111/j.1533-2500.2012.00562.x; Passard A, Attal N, Benadhira R, et al. "Effects of unilateral repetitive transcranial magnetic stimulation of the motor cortex on chronic widespread pain in fibromyalgia." *Brain* 130, no 10 (2007): 2661-70; Leung A, Donohue M, Xu R, et al. "rTMS for suppressing neuropathic pain: A meta-analysis." *Journal of Pain* 10, no. 12 (2009): 1205-16.

Glossary

Acetaminophen   A nonopioid and non-anti-inflammatory pain-relieving medication.

Acupressure   Stimulation of acupuncture points with pressure rather than needles.

Acupuncture   Precise placement of sterilized, hair-thin needles that penetrate the skin to stimulate and rebalance the body's internal energy.

Acute pain   Temporary pain that responds well to medication and dissipates as the body recuperates from an injury or illness.

Alexander technique   A process that relieves muscular tension through recognition of poor postural habits.

Allodynia   Pain resulting from nonpainful stimuli.

Alternative medicine   Therapies that are used instead of conventional Western medical treatment.

Analgesic   A pain-relieving medication.

Anticonvulsant   A medication used to control seizures; also used to reduce neuropathic pain.

Arachnoiditis   A painful condition that develops when the arachnoid membrane surrounding the spinal cord nerves becomes inflamed.

Aromatherapy   The practice of using essential oils to improve psychological and physical well-being.

Arthritis   Inflammation in one or more joints.

Ascending pathways   Nerve pathways that carry sensory information from the spinal cord to the brain.

Aura   A visual disturbance that often precedes migraine headaches.

Autoimmune disease	A condition that develops when a person's immune system attacks healthy tissue.
Ayurvedic medicine	An ancient Indian holistic approach to health.
Beta blocker	A medication that lowers blood pressure and slows the heart rate by blocking adrenaline and noradrenaline (epinephrine and norepinephrine).
Biofeedback	A therapeutic process that trains people to modulate involuntary bodily processes by using deep breathing and other relaxation techniques.
Biologics	Genetically engineered proteins used to treat autoimmune disorders.
Blood patch	A small amount of an individual's blood that is injected into the space surrounding the spinal cord to stop spinal fluid from leaking.
Body mass index (BMI)	The ratio of a person's height to weight.
Bone pain	Severe pain caused by damage to, injury of, or disease in the bone.
Bone spurs	Bumpy growths of new bone that can cause pain.
Botulinum toxin type A (Botox)	A neurotoxic protein used in cosmetic procedures and medical treatments.
Breakthrough pain	Temporary spikes of pain that occur despite medication that otherwise relieves pain.
Bulging disc	A spinal disc that extends beyond its normal space.
Calcium channel blocker	A medication that improves blood flow by decreasing calcium influx into cells.
Capsaicin	The heat-producing ingredient in chili peppers.
Casualgia	A neuropathic pain that typically causes a burning sensation.
Catastrophize	To irrationally believe that something is worse than it is.
Cauda equina syndrome	Extreme compression of nerves in the lower spine.
Cementoplasty	A procedure that injects medical cement into the bone to strengthen and support it.
Central nervous system	The brain and the spinal cord.
Central pain	Disabling pain that originates in the spinal cord or the brain.
Central sensitization	An increased sensitivity to painful or nonpainful stimuli that results when neurons in the brain and the spinal cord become overexcited.
Cerebral cortex	The part of the brain that processes thought.
Cervical facet joints	Spinal joints that facilitate movement of the neck.

Cervical stenosis	Narrowing of the spinal canal or nerve channels in the neck.
Chemoreceptors	Sensory receptors that detect taste, smell, and other chemical changes in the body.
Chiropractic manipulation	Sharp movements made to readjust the spine into proper alignment.
Chronic fatigue syndrome (CFS)	A disorder characterized by debilitating exhaustion that does not improve with adequate rest. It often overlaps with fibromyalgia and other painful conditions.
Chronic pain	Pain that persists after the expected recovery period from an injury or an illness.
Chronic pelvic pain syndrome (CPPS)	A disorder that causes unexplained discomfort at the base of the penis, in the testicles, or in the rectum. (The equivalent in women is referred to as chronic pelvic pain.)
Circadian rhythm	A person's internal body clock that regulates the 24-hour cycle of the biological processes.
Cluster headaches	Bouts of headaches that may occur several times during the day or at the same time each day for several days, weeks, or months.
Cognitive behavioral therapy (CBT)	A type of psychotherapy that helps people change their maladaptive thoughts.
Complementary medicine	Non-Western therapies that are used with conventional treatment.
Complex regional pain syndrome (CRPS)	A type of chronic pain that develops from nerve malfunction.
Congenital analgesia	A rare inherited condition characterized by the inability to feel pain.
Corticosteroid	A natural or manufactured anti-inflammatory hormone.
Cortisol	A naturally produced hormone that is associated with increased stress.
COX-2 inhibitor	A type of anti-inflammatory medication that reduces pain with less risk of gastrointestinal bleeding.
Crepitation	A cracking sound made by arthritic joints.
Deep brain stimulation	A surgical procedure that treats pain and other neurological symptoms that do not respond to medication.
Deep tissue massage	Forceful kneading that releases tension in the deep layers of muscle and connective tissue.
Depression	A persistent state of low motivation, energy, and mood.
Descending pathways	Nerve pathways from the brain to the spinal cord that allow the brain to control bodily functions below the head.
Diabetic neuropathy	Nerve damage caused by diabetes.

Discectomy	Surgery to remove damaged spinal disc material.
Discoplasty	A procedure that uses energy to destroy damaged disc material.
Disease-modifying antirheumatic drugs (DMARDs)	Medications used as a second line of defense to slow the progression of arthritis.
Dorsal horn	The portion of the spinal cord that relays incoming sensations.
Dry-needle procedure	Applying direct pressure to a painful trigger point with an empty syringe.
Dura	The thin membrane surrounding the spinal fluid that covers the brain and the spinal cord.
Electroencephalo-graphy	A type of biofeedback that measures brain-wave activity.
Electromyography	A type of biofeedback that measures muscle tension.
Endocrine system	The body's hormonal system.
Endometriosis	A sometimes painful condition caused when the lining of the uterus spreads beyond the uterus to other areas of the pelvis.
Endorphin	A neurotransmitter released by the brain to reduce pain signals.
Enkephalin	A pain-inhibiting substance that is released by the central nervous system.
Enterovirus	A common virus in the gastrointestinal tract.
Epidural steroid injection	A corticosteroid injection given in the spine but outside the dura, to temporarily reduce inflammation around irritated nerves.
Excitotoxin	A substance that activates neurons in a way that heightens pain sensitivity and damages the neurons.
Extended-release opioid	A pill or patch that slowly releases opioid medication over hours or days.
Facet joint	Spinal joints that control movement between vertebrae.
Facet joint syndrome	Pain caused by injured or arthritic facet joints.
Failed back syndrome	Pain that continues after spinal surgery.
Feldenkrais	A gentle practice that teaches movement with less effort than other exercises.
Fibromyalgia	A chronically painful condition characterized by pain in the joints, muscles, and other soft tissues.
Fight or flight	A biological response that prepares the body to react to a real or perceived threat.
Fluoroscopy	The use of real-time x-ray to guide an injection directly to the targeted area.

Foraminal stenosis	Narrowing of the bony canals where the nerve roots exit the spine.
Gate-Control Theory of pain	The hypothesis that pain pathways are regulated by nerve cells in the spinal cord that act as biological "gates," closing to stop pain signals or opening to let the signals continue to the brain.
General anesthetic	A drug that causes loss of consciousness.
Genetics	The science of heredity.
Genomics	The study of an individual organism's DNA.
Glutamate	A neurotransmitter that facilitates pain signals.
Gout	A type of arthritis that develops from too much uric acid in a single joint, often in the big toe.
Guided imagery	A type of self-induced hypnotic state that is achieved by the use of mental images.
Half-life	The time it takes for the body to clear one-half of a drug.
Herniated disc (also ruptured or slipped disc)	A condition that develops when the gel of a spinal disc protrudes beyond the disc interior.
Herpes zoster infection (shingles)	A painful condition caused by a reactivation of the dormant varicella-zoster virus (the chicken pox virus).
Homeopathic	An alternative medical system based on the belief that highly diluted doses of any substance that produces symptoms can trigger the body's ability to heal itself.
Hyperalgesia	An extraordinary sensitivity to painful stimuli.
Hypersensitivity	An exaggerated bodily response to stimuli.
Hypnosis	A fully conscious trance state characterized by heightened suggestibility and relaxation.
Ibuprofen	A nonsteroidal anti-inflammatory medication.
Ilioinguinal nerve	A nerve that provides sensation to the pubic area and part of the groin.
Immediate-release opioid	An opioid that acts quickly but fades after three to four hours.
Inflammation	The body's immune-system response to injury or irritation.
Inflammatory bowel disease (IBD)	Chronic inflammation of the small intestine (Crohn's disease) or the large intestine (chronic ulcerative colitis).
Intercostal nerves	The system of nerves that supply sensitivity to most of the skin and muscles of the chest and the abdominal wall.

Intradiscal electrothermoplasty	A procedure that relieves disc-related, low-back pain by inserting a heated wire into a spinal disc to destroy pain-causing nerves.
Intrathecal pain pump	A medical device that delivers medications directly into the spinal fluid.
Intravenous immunoglobin	Antibody-replacement therapy produced from donor blood.
Ion channels	Pathways along cell membranes where electrically charged particles enter and exit cells.
Irritable bowel syndrome (IBS)	A chronically painful intestinal disorder that can be difficult to treat.
Jin Shin Jyutsu	A type of massage that uses light pressure on specific body points to release tension and rebalance the body's energies.
Laminotomy or laminectomy	Surgery to remove the bone spurs or part of the vertebra to relieve severe back pain.
Lancinating pain	A stabbing pain.
Laporoscopic spinal fusion	A minimally invasive procedure that joins two discs.
Laughter yoga	A stress-relieving therapy that combines yoga breathing and deliberate laughter.
Lidocaine	A local anesthetic.
Limbic system	Areas of the brain that process smell, behavior, emotion, and emotional association with memory.
Local anesthestic	Medication that numbs painful sensations.
Lumbar endoscopic discectomy	A minimally invasive procedure that destroys or removes damaged disc material.
Lumbar facet joints	Paired joints between and behind the vertebrae of the low back that stabilize the spine and facilitate movement.
Lumbar stenosis	Narrowing of the spinal canal or nerve channels in the lower back.
Lymphedema	Chronic swelling that often develops after radiation therapy or lymph node removal.
Mantra	A word or words that are repeated during meditation.
Mechanoreceptors	Sensory receptors that enable perception of touch, pressure, sounds, and motion (including equilibrium).
Medical marijuana	Leaves or extracts of the cannabis plant that are pre-scribed to relieve chronic symptoms.
Methadone	An opioid-based medication used for moderate to severe pain that does not respond to nonnarcotic analgesics.

Microdiscectomy	A minimally invasive procedure to relieve pain from a herniated disc.
Migraine headaches	Severe pulsing and throbbing head pain that may be preceded by visual disturbances.
Mindfulness	A type of meditation that focuses on the present.
Mirror therapy	Using mirrors to "fool" the brain and treat phantom-limb pain and possibly CRPS.
Morphine	An opiate-based pain medication used to treat moderate-to-severe pain that does not respond to nonnarcotic analgesics.
Moxibustion	Generating heat to acupuncture points by burning a small bundle of herbs.
Myofascial pain	Pain in the muscles.
Myofascial release massage	Kneading that releases tension in the connective tissue.
Myofascial trigger points	Hypersensitive nodules in the muscles and surrounding connecting tissue.
Naproxen sodium	A nonsteroidal anti-inflammatory drug used to relieve pain, inflammation, and fever.
Narcotic	The legal term for a controlled substance.
Naturopathy	A holistic health system that depends on the healing powers of nature.
Nerve	A long fiber-like cell that transfers signals (including sensations) throughout the body (*see* Neurons).
Nerve block	An injection of medication that reduces abnormal firing of sensitive nerves.
Neuralgia	Pain that is caused by damaged or dysfunctional nerves.
Neuritis	Inflammation in one or more nerves.
Neurons	Nerve cells that fire on and off in reaction to chemical and electrical stimuli and act as the body's messenger system.
Neuropathic pain	Pain triggered by an injury or malfunction in the peripheral or the central nervous system that persists after the damaged tissues heal.
Neurostimulator	An implanted device that emits a mild electric current to relieve pain.
Neurotransmitter	A chemical released by nerve cells to carry a signal to the next nerve.
Nocebo effect	A negative response brought about by a negative expectation.
Nociceptive pain	Pain that stems from tissue damage.
Nociceptor	A nerve-cell ending that initiates the sensation of pain.

Nonsteroidal anti-inflammatory drugs (NSAIDs)	A class of pain-reducing medications that also decrease inflammation.
Norepinephrine	A type of neurotransmitter that can decrease pain signals in the spinal cord.
Novocaine	A local anesthetic.
Nucleoplasty	The use of laser or radiofrequency energy to destroy damaged disc material.
Occipital nerves	Nerves that transmit sensation to the back and the top of the head.
Occipital nerve stimulation	Electrical stimulation of the occipital nerve to treat chronic headaches.
Off-label	Use of a medication for a condition that is not included in the FDA's approval.
Opiate	A drug that is derived from opium.
Opioid	A natural or synthetic drug that binds to opioid receptors.
Opioid agonist	A drug that activates mu opioid receptors and mimics endorphins to relieve pain.
Opioid antagonist	A drug that takes up space that would otherwise be used by pain-reducing opioids or endorphins.
Opioid rotation	Changing from one opioid to another to improve a patient's outcome.
Opium	A narcotic from the *Papaver somniferum* poppy.
Osteoarthritis (OA)	Arthritis that develops when joint cartilage progressively deteriorates because of aging.
Osteopathic manipulation	Gently manipulating muscles and joints to relieve pain and stiffness.
Osteoporosis	Thinning of the bones and loss of bone density.
Pain log	A diary of a person's pain experiences.
Pain management	A branch of medicine that uses a multidisciplinary approach to pain relief.
Pain pump	A device that delivers medication directly into the spinal fluid.
Pain specialist	A physician who specializes in the treatment of pain.
Pain threshold	The level of sensory stimulation at which an individual feels pain.
Pain tolerance	The maximum amount of pain an individual is able to withstand.
Paresthesia	An abnormal prickling or burning sensation.
Percutaneous discectomy	A minimally invasive procedure that punctures a ruptured disc to remove damaged disc material.

Peripheral nerves	Nerves outside of the brain and the spinal cord.
Peripheral-nerve stimulation	Using weak electrical current to decrease pain.
Peripheral nervous system	The network of sensory nerve fibers in skin, muscles, and bones that feed information to the spinal cord and the brain.
Peripheral neuropathy	Pain caused by damage to the nerves outside the brain and the spinal cord.
Phantom pain	Pain that is felt in a limb or part of the body that has been removed.
Pharmacogenetics	The study of how an individual's genes affect variations in the response to medication.
Photoreceptors	Sensory receptors that respond to light and enable vision.
Physical therapy	The use of exercise, massage, heat, or other physical modalities to treat disease, injury, or disability.
Physiological	Pertaining to the physical and chemical functions and activities of a living organism.
Pilates	A method of exercise that strengthens core muscles and promotes awareness of posture to lessen spinal stress and tension.
Placebo	A substance with no medical properties.
Placebo effect	A positive response brought about by a positive expectation.
Positive psychology	The study of focusing on aspects that make life worth living.
Positron emission tomography (PET) scan	A noninvasive diagnostic test that produces three-dimensional images of the metabolic activity in the body or the brain.
Postdrome phase	A drowsy, fuzzy sensation that may linger for a day or two after a migraine headache ends.
Postherpetic neuralgia (PHN)	Long-lasting pain from nerve damage caused by shingles.
Postmastectomy pain syndrome	Chronic chest pain that develops when nerves are damaged during mastectomy.
Post-traumatic stress disorder (PTSD)	Severe anxiety caused by physical or emotional trauma.
Premonitory phase (also prodrome phase)	The symptomatic period that precedes a migraine.
Probiotic	Live microorganisms that benefit the digestive system.
Prolotherapy	Using injections of concentrated dextrose to trigger the body's wound-healing response.
Prostaglandins	Chemicals in the body that encourage inflammation and send pain messages to the brain when tissue is injured.

Psychoneuro-immunology	The science of the interdependence between mind and body.
Pulsed radiofrequency	Short bursts of radio energy applied to decrease nerve pain.
Qigong	A Chinese system of slow, gentle movement that includes focused breathing.
Radiofrequency ablation	A procedure that heats nerve tissue with energy to destroy nerves and decrease pain.
Rebound headaches	Headaches caused by frequent use of pain medication.
Referred pain	Pain that is felt at a location other than its point of origin.
Reflexology	The practice of applying pressure to specific points on the feet to stimulate corresponding organs and muscle groups.
Reflex sympathetic dystrophy	A type of chronic pain that develops from nerve malfunction. Now called complex regional pain syndrome (CRPS).
Reiki	Japanese massage therapy that is said to transfer energy from the practitioner to the patient.
Repetitive transcranial magnetic stimulation (rTMS) (also transcranial magnetic stimulation)	Application of noninvasive electromagnetic pulses to the head.
Reuptake	Reabsorption of neurochemicals by the nerves that release them.
Rheumatoid arthritis	A long-term and painful degenerative type of arthritis.
Rheumatologist	A medical professional who specializes in the treatment of arthritis and related diseases.
Rhizotomy	A surgical procedure that deadens nerves to relieve pain.
Rolfing	A type of deep tissue massage.
Sciatica	Pain from pinched or irritated lumbar nerve roots that travel from the spine to the buttock and the leg.
Scoliosis	Curvature of the spine.
Selective serotonin reuptake inhibitors (SSRIs)	The most commonly prescribed class of antidepressants.
Serotonin	A neurotransmitter in the spinal cord that can decrease pain signals.
Serotonin and norepinephrine reuptake inhibitors (SNRIs)	A type of antidepressant medication.

Shiatsu	A Japanese form of acupressure.
Shingles	An extremely painful rash caused by the chicken pox virus.
Somatic pain	Nociceptive pain that affects the skin, muscles, joints, ligaments, or bones.
Spinal headache	A headache caused by leaking spinal fluid.
Spinal stenosis	Narrowing of the spinal canal or nerve channels.
Spinal stimulator	A battery-driven device that delivers a mild electric current to the spinal cord to reduce pain.
Spondylolisthesis	A condition that develops when a vertebra slips out of alignment.
Stump pain	Pain at the site of an amputation.
Substance P	A neurotransmitter released by the central nervous system that creates sensitivity and pain when tissue becomes inflamed or damaged.
Swedish massage	Firm, gentle strokes used to manipulate muscles and connective tissue.
Sympathetic nervous system	Nerves that branch out from the spine and regulate blood flow, sweating, and glandular function.
Synapse	The gap between nerve receptors.
Synovium	The thin membrane lining the joints.
Tai chi	An ancient Chinese regimen that combines slow, graceful physical movement, controlled breathing, and meditation.
Temporomandibular disorders	Jaw pain caused by osteoarthritis, rheumatoid arthritis, or problems in the surrounding muscles or joint.
Tension-type headache	Mild to moderate aching that is often felt to be bandlike around the head.
Thalamus	The part of the brain that processes sensory perception and regulates motor functions.
Thermal biofeedback	A type of biofeedback that measures skin temperature.
Thermoreceptors	Sensory receptors that sense heat, cold, and temperature changes.
Trager Psychophysical Integration	An alternative method of achieving relaxation with passive and active movement.
Transcranial magnetic stimulation (also repetitive transcranial magnetic stimulation)	Application of noninvasive electromagnetic pulses to the head.
Transcutaneous electrical nerve stimulation (TENS) unit	A small device that transmits gentle electrical impulses through the skin to stimulate the nerves and replace painful sensations with a mild tingling.

Transforaminal epidural steroid injection	Injection of a corticosteroid at the spinal exit site of an affected nerve root to treat pain in the lower back or legs.
Tricyclic anti-depressants (TCAs)	The oldest type of medication used to treat depression.
Trigeminal neuralgia	A type of nerve pain in the face that causes a painful burning sensation.
Trigger	A food, behavior, or other influence that activates pain (commonly in reference to headaches).
Trigger-point injection	Local anesthetic administered directly into a painful muscle.
Trigger-point massage	Applying finger pressure to muscles to release tension.
Triptan	A medication developed specifically to abort migraine headaches.
Tui na	A type of alternative massage that emphasizes rebalancing and restoration of the body's energy.
Visceral pain	Pain that involves the internal organs.
Yoga	An ancient Indian discipline that combines physical postures, breathing, and meditation.

Resources

Pain Organizations

American Academy of Hospice and Palliative Medicine (www.aahpm.org)

American Academy of Pain Medicine (www.painmed.org)

The American Cancer Society (www.cancer.org)

American Chronic Pain Association (www.theacpa.org)

American Pain Society (www.ampainsoc.org)

Americans for Better Care for the Dying (www.abcd-caring.org)

For Grace: Empowering Women in Pain (www.forgrace.org)

International Association for the Study of Pain (www.iasp-pain.org)

The Mayday Pain Project (www.painandhealth.org)

The National Women's Health Information Center (www.womenshealth.gov)

Pain.com (www.pain.com)

Partners against Pain (www.partnersagainstpain.com)

U.S. Pain Foundation (uspainfoundation.org)

Support Organizations for Specific Conditions

American Back Society (www.americanbacksoc.org)

American College of Rheumatology (www.rheumatology.org)

American Council for Headache Education (www.achenet.org)

American Headache Society (www.americanheadachesociety.org)

American Migraine Foundation (www.americanmigrainefoundation.org)

The Arthritis Foundation (www.arthritis.org)

Cancer Care (www.cancercare.org)

Crohn's & Colitis Foundation of America (www.ccfa.org)

The Hubbard Foundation (www.hubbardfoundation.org)

IBD Support Foundation (www.ibdsf.com)

International Foundation for Functional Gastrointestinal Disorders (www.iffgd
.org)

Mesothelioma Cancer Alliance (www.mesothelioma.com)

National Fibromyalgia & Chronic Pain Association (www.fmcpaware.org)

National Fibromyalgia Association (www.fmaware.org)

National Headache Foundation (www.headaches.org)

National Shingles Foundation (www.vzvfoundation.org)

National Vulvodynia Association (www.nva.org)

Patient Alliance for Neuroendocrineimmune Disorders Organization for
Research and Advocacy (www.pandoraorg.net)

Reflex Sympathetic Dystrophy Syndrome Association (www.rsds.org)

The Spinal Research Foundation (www.spinerf.org)

Spine Universe (www.spineuniverse.com)

The TMJ Association (www.tmj.org)

The Vulvar Pain Foundation (www.thevpfoundation.org)

Clinical Trials

ClinicalTrials.gov (www.clinicaltrials.gov)

Index

Page numbers in *italics* indicate figures and tables.

back pain. *See* low-back pain
beta blockers, 75, 210
biofeedback, 93-95, 210, 219
biologics, 25, 210
blood patches, 37, 210
body mass index (BMI), 104, 210
body-over-pain therapies: destruction
    of nerves and tissue, 125-26; exercise,
    98-101; injections, implants, and
    neurostimulators, 113-15, *115, 116,*
    117-25, *118,* 122; intradiscal proce-
    dures, 126-28; nutrition and diet,
    105-11; passive physical therapies,
    101-3; weight loss, 103-5
bone pain, 210
bone spurs, 21, 210
Botox, 35, 210
brain: cerebral cortex, 15-16, 210; cingu-
    late cortex, 86; deep brain stimulation,
    124-25, 211; Gate-Control Theory, 7-8;
    nociceptors and, 16; pathways to and
    from, 6-7, *7,* 9-11; thalamus, 15, 219.
    See also neurotransmitters
breakthrough pain, 61, 210
breathing to reduce stress, 95, 96
bulging discs, 38, *38,* 210
buprenorphine, 60-61, *63*

caffeine and headaches, 30-31
calcium, 111-12, 113
calcium channel blockers, 75, 210
CAM. *See* complementary and alternative
    medicine
cancer pain, 26-27, 51
cannabinoids, 76-77
capsaicin, 73, 210
capsaicin skin cream (Zostrix), 22
carbamazepine (Tegretol, Carbatrol), 71
casualgia, 210
catastrophizing, 80, 210
categorizing pain, 3-5
cauda equina syndrome, 40, 210
CBT (cognitive behavioral therapy),
    88-89, 211

celecoxib (Celebrex), 58-59
cementoplasty, 26, 210
central nervous system, 6, 210
central sensitization, 9, 28, 210
cerebral cortex, 15-16, 210
cervical facet joint pain, 42, 210
cervical stenosis, *39,* 39-40, 211
CFS (chronic fatigue syndrome), 49-50, 211
chemoreceptors, 211
children, impact of pain on, 172-73
Chinese acupuncture, 133
chiropractic manipulation, 103, 211
chronic fatigue syndrome (CFS), 49-50, 211
chronic pain: acute pain compared to, *2;*
    consequences of, xvii; described, 2-3,
    211; forms of, xvii; as global problem,
    190; myths about, 4-5. *See also* body-
    over-pain therapies; complementary
    and alternative medicine; conditions,
    chronically painful; management of
    pain; medications for pain; mind-over-
    pain therapies
chronic pelvic pain syndrome, 211
chronic ulceritis, 49
cingulate cortex, 86
circadian rhythm, 34, 211
clinical trials, 131, 222
clonazepam (Klonopin, Rivotril), 71
cluster headaches, 31, 211
cognitive behavioral therapy (CBT),
    88-89, 211
combat injuries, 18-19
combined nociceptive and neuropathic
    pain, 4, *5*
communication: among family members,
    170, 172-73, 174-75; with physicians,
    184-85
complementary and alternative medicine
    (CAM): energy-based therapies, 131-36;
    holistic and nature-based therapies,
    140-48; mind-body movements, 136-40;
    overview of, 129-31, 211; in U.S., *130*
complex regional pain syndrome (CRPS):
    analgesics for, 74; case examples,

100-101, 176-77, 188-89; described, 43-44, 211; nerve blocks and, 115, 117-18; NMDA-receptor antagonists and, 72

computer headaches, 36

conditions, chronically painful: cancer, 26-27, 51; chronic fatigue syndrome, 49-50; headaches, 29-37; inflammatory bowel disease, 49; irritable bowel syndrome, 48; low-back and neck pain, 37-43, *38*; myofascial pain, 45-46; pelvic pain, 46-47; phantom pain, 47-48; postoperative pain, 2, 50-51; shingles, 9, 44-45. *See also* arthritis; complex regional pain syndrome; fibromyalgia

congenital analgesia, 1, 211

control, taking: diagnosis and treatment, 180-83; facing fears, 179-80; living well, 185-89; physician appointments, 183-85, *184*

corticosteroids, 23, 73-74, 211

cortisol, 92, 137, 211

cost of treatments and lost productivity, xviii

Cousins, Norman, 96-97

COX-2 inhibitors, *58*, 58-59, 211

crepitation, 21, 211

Crohn's disease, 49

CRPS. *See* complex regional pain syndrome

da Vinci, Leonardo, 6

deep brain stimulation, 124-25, 211

deep breathing, 95

deep tissue massage, 102, 211

degenerative joint disease, 22-23

delivery of pain medication, 193

Depakote ER, Depakene (valproic acid), 71

dependence on opioids, 66-68

depression: antidepressants, 12, 69-70; case example, 81-82; confronting, 80-81; described, 211

Descartes, René, 7-8

descending pathway to brain, 7, 211

describing pain, 185, *186*

devil's claw, 142

diabetes and diabetic neuropathy, 43, 211

diagnosis, 180, 182-83

diaries: food, 111; headache, 30, 33; journaling in, 97, 164; pain logs, 216

diet and nutrition, 105-13. *See also* triggers

dietary supplements, 141-44

Dilantin (phenytoin), 71

direct chemoreceptors, *12*

disc damage and low-back pain, *38*, 38-40, 126-28

discectomy, 212

discoplasty, 127, 212

disease-modifying antirheumatic drugs (DMARDs), 24-25, 212

distant chemoreceptors, *12*

dopamine, 195

dorsal horn, 6, *10*, 212

double-blind, placebo-controlled studies, 131

dry-needle procedure, 212

dura, 37, 212

education, pain as, 154-55

electroencephalography, 212

electromyography, 212

emotion: facing fears, 179-80; helplessness, 173; pain as, 78; stress as heightening pain, 79-82, *81*; unhealthy, in family with chronic pain, *169*

endocrine system, 27, 212

end-of-life pain, 27

endometriosis, 46, 212

endorphins, 12, 13-15, 212

endoscopic laminotomy, 127-28

energy-based therapies: acupressure, 134-35; acupuncture, 131-34; magnets, 135-36; reflexology, 135; Reiki, 135

enkephalin, 212

enteroviruses, 49, 212

epidural steroid injections, *118*, 118-19, 212

ergotamines, 35

estrogen and pain perception, 17-18

ethnic minorities and pain, 19-20
excitotoxin, 212
exercise, 98-101
expectations, altering, 85-86
experience and perception of pain, 16
extended-release opioids, 212

facet joints, 212
facet joint syndrome, 212
failed back syndrome, 212
family dynamics: action plan for, 174-77; case example, 176-77; impact of pain on children, 172-73; impact of pain on spouse or partner, 170-72; overview of, 168, 170; reinforcement of pain and sabotage of recovery, 173-74; unhealthy emotions, *169*
fats, 106-8
fears, facing, 179-80
feelings. *See* emotion
Feldenkrais, 140, 212
fentanyl, 60, 61, *63*
feverfew, 142
fibromyalgia: diet and, 108; magnesium and, 113; overview of, 27-29, 212; substance P and, 11; tai chi and, 138-39; yoga and, 137-38
fight-or-flight response, 92, 212
fluoroscopy, 212
focused meditation, 88
food triggers, 110-11
foraminal stenosis, 43, 213
Frankl, Victor, 156

gabapentin (Neurontin), 70-71
gamma-amino butyric acid, 11
gamma linolenic acid, 143
Gate-Control Theory, 7-8, 213
gender: perception of pain and, 17-18; response to opioids and, 68
general anesthetic, 213
genetics: defined, 213; discoveries and trends in, 193-94; testing for medication effectiveness and, 62

genomics, 213
ginger, 142-43
giving to others, 166
glucosamine and chondroitin, 23, 143
glutamate, 11, 72, 213
gout, 25-26, 108-9, 213
gratitude, cultivating, 163-66
guided imagery, 90-91, 213

half-life, 213
hasya (laughter yoga), 97, 214
hatha yoga, forms of, 137
headaches: cluster, 31, 211; computer, 36; migraine, *32*, 32-35, 94-95, 110, 112-13, 215; overview of, 29-30; rebound, 31-32, 218; spinal, 37, 219; tension-type, 35-37, 219
health care system, xi-xii, 190-91
health insurance and CAM therapies, 148
help, asking for, 176
helplessness, reinforcement of, 173
herbal therapies, 141-44, 148
herniated discs, *38*, 38-39, 118, 213
herpes zoster infection (shingles), 9, 44-45, 213
holistic and nature-based therapies: aromatherapy, 144-46, 209; Ayurvedic medicine, 147-48, 210; herbs and nutritional supplements, 141-44; homeopathy, 146-47, 213; naturopathy, 147, 215; overview of, 140-41
homeopathy, 146-47, 213
humor, 95-97
Huo Luo Xiao Ling Dan, 144
hydrocodone (Vicodin), 31
hydromorphone, *63*
hyperalgesia, 64, 213
hypersensitivity, 213
hypnosis, 89-90, 213

ibuprofen, 57, *58*, 213
ignoring pain, 8-9
ilioinguinal nerve, 117, 213
immediate-release opioids, 213

immune system, 23-24, 91, 210

implantable/intrathecal pain pumps, 119-20, 214, 216

inflammation, 213

inflammatory bowel disease, 49, 213

injections, 114-15, *116*, 117-19, 212, 220

Institute of Medicine, *Relieving Pain in America,* xvii-xviii

integrative medicine, 196

intercostal nerves, 117, 213

interpretation of pain, 78-79

intimacy and pain, 171-72

intradiscal procedures, 126-28, 214

intravenous immunoglobulin (IVIG), 74, 214

ion channels, 193, 214

irritable bowel syndrome, 48, 109, 214

IVIG (intravenous immunoglobulin), 74, 214

Japanese acupuncture, 133

Jin Shin Jyutsu, 135, 214

journaling, 97, 164

Kabat-Zinn, John, 89

kappa receptors, targeting with medication, 192-93

ketamine, 72-73

Klonopin (clonazepam), 71

laminectomy, 127, 214

lancinating pain, 214

laporoscopic spinal fusion, 214

laughter yoga (hasya), 97, 214

lidocaine, 72, 214

limbic system, 16, 214

living well with pain, 185-89

local anesthetics, 72, 214

low-back pain: disc damage and, *38,* 38-40, 118; lumbar facet joint pain, 40-41; nerve damage, 41-42; overview of, 37-38

lumbar endoscopic discectomy, 127, 214

lumbar facet joint pain, 40-41, 214

lumbar stenosis, *39, 39-40,* 214

lymphedema, 51, 214

Lyrica (pregabalin), 71

magnesium, 112-13

magnets, 135-36

managed care system, 190-91

management of pain: endorphin levels and, 12; as priority, 187; tools for, *188*; trends in, 191-96; as trial-and-error process, 186-87. *See also* medications for pain; treatment

mantra meditation, 88, 214

marijuana, medical, 76-77, 214

meaning of pain, 153-55

mechanics of pain, 5-9

mechanoreceptors, *12,* 214

medical marijuana, 76-77

medications for pain: acetaminophen, 53-54, *54*; adjunct, for neuropathic pain, 68-73; alcohol, mixing with, 59; analgesics, 4, 18, 23, 52-53, 73-77; anesthetics, 72; anticonvulsants, 70-71; antidepressants, 12, 69-70; clinical trials of, 76; expectations for, 85-86; management of, 53; methadone, 31, 60; NMDA-receptor antagonists, 72-73; off-label, 216; overview of, 52-53; prediction of response to, 62; tolerance for, 66-67; trends in, 191-93. *See also* nonsteroidal anti-inflammatory drugs; opioids

meditation: mindful, 87, 89, 161, 215; myths about, *88*; prayer as, 159; spiritual, 160-61; types of, 88

Melzack, Ronald, 8

memantine, 73

methadone: for pain, 60, *63,* 214; for rebound headaches, 31

microdiscectomy, 127, 215

migraine headaches: biofeedback for, 94-95; described, 32-35, 215; food triggers for, 110; magnesium and, 112-13; ordinary headaches compared to, *32* mind-body movements: Pilates, 139-40; tai chi and qigong, 138-39; yoga, 136-38

mind-body process: placebo response, 13-15; psychoneuroimmunology, 91

mindful meditation, 87, 89, 161, 215

mind-over-pain therapies: changing thinking, 82-92; overview of, 78-79; stress as heightening pain, 79-82, *80*, *81*; stress management and relaxation tools, 92-97

minorities and pain, 19-20

mirror therapy, 47-48, 215

monosodium glutamate (MSG), 110-11

morphine, 59, *63,* 215

motivation to engage life, 156-57, 158

movement meditation, 88

moxibustion, 131, 215

MSG (monosodium glutamate), 110-11

mucuna pruriens, 148

multidisciplinary therapies, 180, 196

muscle relaxants, 75

myofascial pain, 45-46, 215

myofascial release massage, 102, 215

myofascial trigger points, 132, 215

myths about chronic pain, 4-5

naloxone, 14

naproxen sodium, 215

narcotics, 60, 215

naturopathy, 147, 215

neck pain, 42-43

negative thinking: catastrophizing, 79-80; impact of, *80*; reframing, *89*. *See also* thoughts, changing

nerve blocks, 114-15, *115, 116,* 117-19, 215

nerves: described, 215; destruction of, 125-26; spinal, damage to, 41-42; stimulation of, 121, 122-24; types of, 117, 213, 216, 217. *See also* nerve blocks

neuralgia, 215

neuritis, 215

neurons, 9, *10, 11,* 215

Neurontin (gabapentin), 70-71

neuropathic pain: adjunct medications for, 68-73; conditions leading to, *5*; described, 3-4, 215; medications for, 28

neuropathy, 43

neurostimulators, 121-25, *122*, 195-96, 215

neurotransmitters: described, 215; examples of, 11-12; in pathway to brain, 9-11; regulation and replacement of, 195. *See also* serotonin

NMDA-receptor antagonists, 72-73

N-methyl-D-aspartate (NMDA) receptors, 60

nocebo effect, 68, 85, 215

nociceptive pain: conditions leading to, *5*; described, 3, 215; neuropathic pain compared to, 4

nociceptors, 3, 215

nonsteroidal anti-inflammatory drugs (NSAIDs): aspirin, *56,* 56-57; COX-2 inhibitors, *58,* 58-59, 211; ibuprofen, 57, *58,* 213; osteoarthritis and, 22; overview of, 54-56, 216

norepinephrine, 11-12

novocaine, 216

NSAIDs. *See* nonsteroidal anti-inflammatory drugs

nucleoplasty, 127, 216

nutritional supplements, 141-44

nutrition and diet, 105-13. *See also* triggers

obesity and pain, 103-5

occipital nerves, 117, 216

occipital nerve stimulation, 123-24, 216

off-label, 216

older adults, chronic pain in, 18

omega-3 fats, 106-7

open discectomy, 126-27

opiates, 216

opioid agonists, 216

opioid antagonists, 216

opioid rotation, 216

opioids: controversy, underuse, and misunderstanding of, 64-66; dependence

pulsed radiofrequency, 126, 218
pumps, implantable/intrathecal, 119-20,
  214, 216
punishment, pain as, 154

qigong, 138-39, 218

RA. *See* rheumatoid arthritis
racial minorities and pain, 19-20
radiofrequency nerve ablation, 125-26, 218
rebound headaches, 31-32, 218
referred pain, 45, 218
reflexology, 135, 218
reflex sympathetic dystrophy. *See* complex regional pain syndrome
reframing thoughts. *See* thoughts,
  changing
Reiki, 135, 218
Relieving Pain in America (Institute of Medicine), xvii-xviii
religion, spirituality compared to, 150-51
repetitive joint stress, 22
repetitive transcranial magnetic stimulation, 125, 195-96, 218
resources, 221-22
reuptake, 69, 218
rheumatoid arthritis (RA): genetics and,
  193-94; omega-3 fats and, 107; overview
  of, 23-25, 218; substance P and, 11
rheumatologists, 22, 24, 218
rhizotomy, 218
rituals, 162, *162*
Rolfing Structural Integration, 102, 218
RSD. *See* complex regional pain syndrome

safety of CAM therapies, 130-31, 148
sciatica, 41, 42, 218
science of pain: categorizing pain, 3-5;
  mechanics of pain, 5-9; overview of, 1-3
scoliosis, 218
scope of problem, xviii
secondary gains, 173-74
selective serotonin reuptake inhibitors
  (SSRIs), 70, 218

Seligman, Martin, 91-92
sensory receptors, *12*
serotonin, 11-12, 34, 195, 218
serotonin and norepinephrine reuptake
  inhibitors (SNRIs), 69-70, 218
Shiatsu, 134, 219
shingles, 9, 44-45, 213, 219
side effects: of NSAIDs, 55-56; of opioids,
  63-64
sleep and exercise, 100
SNRIs (serotonin and norepinephrine
  reuptake inhibitors), 69-70, 218
social withdrawal, 175-76
somatic pain, 3, 219
spinal cord stimulators, 121-22, 219
spinal headaches, 37, 219
spinal manipulation, 103
spinal pumps, implantable/intrathecal,
  119-20, 214, 216
spirituality: case example, 166-67;
  meaning of pain, 153-55; overview
  of, 149-51; pain compared to suffering,
  152-53; resources for, 167; response to
  pain and, xiii; tools to move beyond
  pain, 155-67
spiritual meditation, 88
spondylolisthesis, 42, 219
spouse, impact of pain on, 170-72
SSRIs (selective serotonin reuptake inhibitors), 70, 218
Stavzor (valproic acid), 71
stem cell therapy, 194
stenosis, spinal, *39,* 39-40, 219
stress, as heightening pain, 79-82, *81*
stress management and relaxation tools:
  biofeedback, 93-95; deep breathing, 95;
  humor, 95-97; journaling, 97; laughter
  yoga, 97; overview of, 92-93; progressive muscle relaxation, 93
stump pain, 219
substance P, 11-12, 193, 219
suffering, pain compared to, 152-53
support for partner in pain, 171
support groups, 189

support organizations, 221-22
Swedish massage, 102, 219
sympathetic nervous system, 115, 219
synapses, 9, *10*, 219
synovium, 24, 219

tai chi, 138-39, 219
tapentadol, *63*
TCAs (tricyclic antidepressants), 69, 220
Tegretol (carbamazepine), 71
temporomandibular disorders, 132-33, 219
TENS (transcutaneous electrical nerve stimulation), 121, 219
tension-type headaches, 35-37, 219
tetrahydrocannabinol (THC), 76
thalamus, 15, 219
therapeutic massage, 102
thermal/temperature biofeedback, 93, 219
thermoreceptors, *12*, 219
thoughts: negative, 79-80, *80, 89*; positive, 67-68. *See also* thoughts, changing
thoughts, changing: case examples, 83-85; cognitive behavioral therapy, 88-89; expectations, 85-86; guided imagery, 90-91; hypnosis, 89-90; meditation, 88, *88*; mindful meditation, 87; overview of, 82-83; positive psychology, 91-92; spiritual thoughts, 155-56, *156*
tissue, destruction of, 125-26
TMS. *See* repetitive transcranial magnetic stimulation
tolerance for medication, 66-67
topiramate (Topamax), 71
traction, 40
Trager Psychophysical Integration, 103, 140, 219
training for health care workforce, xii
tramadol (Ultram), 73
transcranial magnetic stimulation. *See* repetitive transcranial magnetic stimulation
transcutaneous electrical nerve stimulation (TENS), 121, 219
trans fats, 107-8

transforaminal epidural steroid injections, 118, 220
treatment: to close pain gates, 8; cost of, xviii; multidisciplinary, 180, 196; by primary physicians, xviii. *See also* body-over-pain therapies; complementary and alternative medicine; management of pain; medications for pain; mind-over-pain therapies
tricyclic antidepressants (TCAs), 69, 220
trigeminal neuralgia, 220
trigger-point injections, 46, 220
trigger-point massage, 102, 220
triggers: food allergies and, 110-11; for headaches, 30, 34, 35, 110; for pain, 220
Trileptal (oxcarbazepine), 71
triptans, 35, 220
Tui na, 135, 220
turmeric, 143
turning pain on or off, 86

Ultram (tramadol), 73
ultrasound, 101
uric acid and gout, 25

valproic acid (Depakote ER, Depakene, Stavzor), 71
value assigned to pain, 16
veterans, military, perceptions of pain in, 18-19
Vicodin (hydrocodone), 31
visceral pain, 3, 220
vitamin D, 111-12, 113

Wall, Patrick, 8
weight loss, 103-5
women, chronic pain in, 17-18
World Health Organization, xvii
writing, as therapy, 97. *See also* diaries

yoga, 136-38, 220

ziconotide (Prialt), 75
Zostrix (capsaicin skin cream), 22

About the Authors

Steven H. Richeimer, M.D., is a preeminent voice in the field of pain management. Passionate about supporting and improving the lives of patients and families affected by chronic pain, he has helped thousands live more productive lives. Board certified in pain medicine, anesthesiology, and psychiatry, Dr. Richeimer is chief of the Division of Pain Medicine at the University of Southern California. He is also director of Pain Management at Norris Cancer Hospital, Los Angeles, and associate professor, Departments of Anesthesiology and Psychiatry, University of Southern California.

Kathy Steligo is the author of *The Breast Reconstruction Guidebook* and co-author of *Confronting Hereditary Breast and Ovarian Cancer*.